International Society For Contact Lens Research

International Society For Contact Lens Research

The First 30 years

Raymond I. Myers, OD

Co-Founder, International Society for Contact Lens Research

Clinical Professor, University of Missouri—St. Louis

Library of Congress Control Number: 2009905244
ISBN: Hardcover   978-1-4415-3914-4
               Softcover   978-1-4415-3913-7

The front cover includes a depiction of "Tree of Knowledge", a memorial to Otto Wichterle next to the Institute of Macromolecular Chemistry in Prague, Czechoslovakia. Each branch of the "Tree" represents a patent of Dr. Wichterle, including a 1941 patent for nylon developed during Nazi occupation of Czechoslovakia in 1938, to multiple patents for the hydrophilic contact lens. The monument was created in 2005 by artists Michal Gabriel, Oleg Haman and Jana Podpěrová. The photograph was taken by Ivan Pinkava, head of the Studio of Photography at the Academy of Arts, Architecture and Design in Prague. Myers gratefully acknowledges Director Frantisek Rypácek of the Institute for his assistance.

This book was printed in the United States of America.

To order additional copies of this book, contact:
Xlibris Corporation
1-888-795-4274
www.Xlibris.com
Orders@Xlibris.com
60149

Contents

Introduction

I have been persuaded by the ISCLR Executive Council to tell the story of the International Society for Contact Lens Research which is about an organization that has been a center of active interchange for many of its members. The Board's direction was to develop a chronology of events and people that have kept it a vibrant for 30 years. A wealth of research material exists because the Proceedings, Programs, Minutes and Constitutions are available from its history on the ISCLR Website(www.ISCLR.org).

The International Society for Contact Lens Research was formed in 1978 for the purpose of uniting various disciplines and regions of the world where the new flexible soft lens field caused separate and divergent pathways of development. There were great expectations of widespread acceptance starting in 1960 (Wichterle O. L., 1960) with the publication of Wichterle and Lim's patent on hydrogels. How that would occur remained uncertain, because new challenges in optics, physiology, and microbiology clearly demonstrated that the full potential of hydrogels would take time to develop.

The ISCLR has played an inordinate role in these developments because its small organization brought together major researchers and manufacturers every two years to assess the field and consider its future direction. Also, the ISCLR invested a significant amount of their resources in bringing individuals from related fields who could contribute to the problems of the time. There was a concerted effort to bring graduate level research students that not only inspired their development, but the students more quickly became the next generation of contact lens researchers and ISCLR leaders. In the space of 30 years, the ISCLR has had presidents representing three generations of leaders.

ISCLR has played a major role in leading the contact lens field into multiple disciplines that have contributed today to a complex, scientific field. Time and again, new researchers came to ISCLR Symposia, made their contributions, learned at the meeting how their interests were connected; and became members or extended their research to contact lenses.

The ISCLR is rich with "characters" that have contributed their knowledge, humor, and sacrifice. The Society's patron Otto Wichterle was a dissident politically and professionally. He not only invented the hydrogels lens material, but found himself proselytizing to groups outside of polymer chemistry who initially found the concept of a flexible lens anathema to the optical precision of a rigid contact lens or ophthalmic lens. At ISCLR meetings, members recounted his enthusiasm and dynamism although in his home country of Czechoslovakia he was held back most of his career by repressive political systems. Montague Ruben, a cofounder and first president, straddled between ophthalmology and optometry as the most recognized individual in the contact field at ISCLR's inception. Being an ophthalmologist in a predominantly optometric field was an extraordinarily difficult tight rope for which his ISCLR contributions required great ingenuity. Co founder Brien Holden, whose enormous contributions included a dedication to ISCLR, spanned more than a quarter century. There is a mythology, not entirely limited to Holden, which built up among these individuals whose accomplishments were only exceeded by their sense of humor!

Members have considered ISCLR as particularly important in providing a direction to the contact lens community as well as personally among their most rewarding meetings. In its existence there have been 216 members through 2007, with 87 charter members. At least 68 charter members remained for at least 10 years, and another 23 are still members today.

I gratefully acknowledge the significant assistance I gained from a variety of members and organizations without which the book and its photos could not have been written. In addition, a group of ISCLR members contributed their writings and insights to this volume. A special thanks goes to Brien Holden who as the author of the Postscript performs his unceasing role with ISCLR as its seer and provocateur. Also, Dwight Cavanagh communicated the insight of the Board why I should undertake this challenge. Others include: Perry Binder, Nathan Efron, Brien Holden, Stephen Klyce, Kenneth Polse, Miguel Refojo, and Deborah Sweeney. At various stages many have contributed to finding the photos, and critiquing the manuscript. In particular, the 2007 Executive Committee and particularly Suzanne Fleiszig, Philip Morgan, and Michel Guillon; Roger Buckley, John Dart, Paul Erickson, Antonio Henriquez, Joshua Josephson, Peter Fanti, Charles McMonnies, Jerry Paugh, Richard Pearson, and Geoffrey Woodward.

My co-worker is Ms. Naadei Nikoi, a UM-St. Louis College of Optometry student whose previous archival experience at Baylor University enabled her to compile and digitize the ISCLR archives from which the book could be referenced.

I also recognize organizations who have contributed research assistance in these efforts including the University of Missouri-St. Louis; Institute of Macromolecular Chemistry in Prague; Czechoslovakia, Moorfields Eye Hospital of London; International Archives, Library, and Museum of Optometry of St. Louis, Missouri; and the British Contact Lens Association of London.

Chapter 1

Contact Lenses in the 1970's

Before Hydrogels and PMMA

The concept of contact lenses occurred as early as Leonardo DaVinci in 1508 where he conceived the idea of changing the refractive surface but his drawings did not represent a practical application.

Rene Descartes in 1637 and Sir John Herschel in 1845 presented other theoretical aspects without actually placing a lens on the eye. (Ruben, Soft Contact Lenses: Clinical and Applied Technology, 1978) (Phillips & Speedwell, 2007)

The availability of materials such as glass, acrylic, and later polymethyl methacrylate allowed for an optically clear and workable material that could be modified to the shape of the cornea and the lids. Thomas Young Muller in the 1887 used blown glass to place a lens with the effect of restoring some vision on diseased eyes.

PMMA Lenses

Polymethyl methacrylate (PMMA) was developed, and its formability and machinability made it useful first with scleral lenses and later with corneal contact lenses. William Feinbloom in 1936 used PMMA as a scleral contact lens, and Theodore Obrig produced the first corneal contact lens in 1938. Corneal contact lenses flourished during the 1960's with a significant degree of acceptance throughout the world. Although there were significant limitations in the numbers of individuals who would achieve full time comfort, many refractive errors were correctable and lens parameters were manipulated, from lens size, curvatures, and thicknesses to achieve acceptable physiological response. Irregular corneas, disfigured eyes, and aphakia provided medical indications which extended its benefit beyond cosmesis.

A familiarity with the hard lens field is important to contrast the changes that would occur with hydrophilic lenses. Hard lens fitting and manufacturing were highly technical because PMMA, when machine forming a specific relationship of the eye, was inflexible and required precise reproduction to maintain good physiology and comfort. Tolerances were very small—hundredths of a millimeter with curvatures and thicknesses: to establish good lens optics, lens movement, and lens positioning. Each practitioner could design the best fitting lens specific for the eye, perhaps using trial lenses to gain an initial impression of fit. Manufacturers then produced each lens uniquely using precise lathing techniques. Lenses were durable, although they scratched easily, and many practitioners developed modification techniques either to polish the lenses or make subtle fitting changes. Corneal physiology was a consideration because the hard lens changed the corneal curvature and the surrounding ocular tissues.

The precision equipment for PMMA came from other manufacturing purposes and were, developed in small companies in innovative ways to both manufacturer lenses as well as to produce specialized special lenses such as bifocals and torics. Jewelry lathes were commonplace in the 1960's along with adaptations of a range of products: polishing compounds used for metals (e.g., Silvo), sponge-like tools from the drug store shelf(Eg., Dr. Scholl's footpads). Line bifocals initially could also be produced by the practitioners through covering half the anterior surface with finger nail polish, and changing the power of the other half with a rotating "toe pad" tool or drum tool.

Considerable research surrounding corneal and lid physiology, and optics were conducted by impressive groups of researchers including the University of California and the Ohio State University Colleges of Optometry. Moorfields Eye Hospital in London developed a large medical department for scleral and corneal contact lenses which included a specialized manufacturing facility.

Otto Wichterle

Wichterle's character, scientific integrity, and prominence as inventor, makes him the appropriate "patron" to the International Society for Contact Lenses. The development of a new approach to contact lenses came from an unlikely place, a satellite communist country, albeit an established reputation before World War 2, where hard lenses were practically unknown. A Czechoslovakian chemist invented the contact lens material in mid 1955 with a hydrophilic plastic material with potential biocompatibility for many uses.

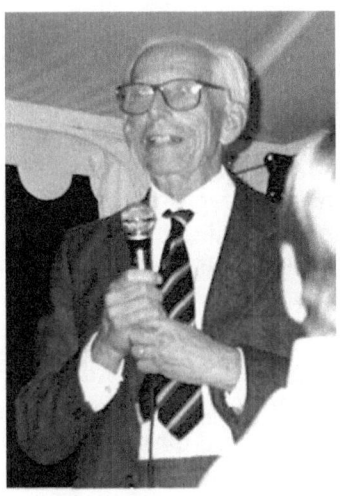

Otto Wichterle, inventor of the hydrophilic lens

Otto Wichterle was associated with the Macromolecular Institute in Prague when he discovered a copolymer material that would eventually produce a hydrophilic, flexible, optically clear, and stable material. Drahoslov Lim was a young colleague who worked with him during early development. The first announcements of the material and subsequent patent described a material that could be used within the body, as a bandage on the skin, as well as a contact lens. In the ensuing ten years, he tested contact lenses initially with spin cast and later lathe-cut manufacturing technology, and clinically worked with the ophthalmologist Maximilian Dreifus.

He achieved international prominence in 1960 for this material defined by a patent and an article in *Nature*. (Wichterle O. L., 1960) This caused a furor of interest in countries that resulted in invitations to present data at scientific gatherings throughout the world. He found many skeptics, especially among the traditional hard lens manufacturers. Considering the preciseness of hard lens manufacturing and the power effects of rigid lenses, it took time to understand that a flexible material would produce the optical precision on the eye. Those within hard contact lens manufacturing were perhaps the furthest from accepting the theoretical possibilities for this new paradigm (Koetting, 1990).

Individuals as well as corporations also visited him in Prague. One of the earliest was Martin Pollak of National Patent Development Corporation (NPDC), representing a small American corporation looking for licensing technology in the east bloc. They quickly were granted worldwide rights through Wichterle and the Czechoslovakian government. Also, Allen Eisen, OD, Robert Morrison,

OD, and Bausch & Lomb became interested in the technology. Bausch & Lomb was early and furnished the capital and R&D necessary for developing spin casting for which NPDC granted them world rights. Spin cast lenses came out first because the first lenses were molded and could not be machined in dry form or after the lens had been polymerized. Wichterle's association with many professionals and hard lens manufacturers, particularly George Nissel in 1963 recognized the attractiveness of using traditional hard lens technology. NPDC was free to market and sublicense the lathe cut lens, referred to as the xerogel material which Wichterle developed later.

Wichterle's role cannot be confined to his invention of the material, but includes all elements of recognizing its potential, conducting or collaborating in biomedical and clinical testing in Czechoslovakia, advocating for its use, and producing the first lenses that were parsed to a few researchers throughout the world. Richard Hill expressed his recollections of Wichterle. "I first met Professor Otto Wichterle at a meeting in Chicago in the 1960's," says Hill. "In the course of our discussion, he gave me one of his unhydrated HEMA buttons, which remains a treasured memento of that age." When the communist Czechoslovakia government would not allow him to develop an applied application at the Macromolecular Institute, he brought the project home on a Christmas vacation. Using his son's "Erector Set," he produced the first generation of a spin casting machine. For several generations of machines, he produced contact lenses that were used for clinical purposes, some were tested in studies in Prague, and others were sent around the world.

Wichterle lived in Czechoslovakia from his birth in 1913 to his death in 1998, and throughout his life he achieved great accomplishments amid major adversities (Wichterle O., Recollections, 1994). During his productive life, Czechoslovakia was occupied by the Nazis in the late 1930's and 1940's, and later in two occupations by Russia in 1960-80's. Born of a prominent capitalist family, he was identified both as an activist in the scientific community, a brilliant scientist, and administrator when he was not up against the establishment. Wichterle's own submission of a biographical sketch to the International Optical Year Book in the early 1980's is testament to his character and range of accomplishments. See Appendix 9. He presents his life events with a brutal honesty such as to state in a few words, "Expelled," "Gestapo Prison,1942-43," "Member, Czechoslovak Federal Parliament" during the Alexander Dubcek government between years of communist rule(International Optical Year Book and Diary, 1983 & 1994).

In 1989 Russian control of the Czechoslovakia suddenly ended before the fall of the Soviet Union. Again, Wichterle was prominent, when he described himself as a "pensioner." He was elected President of the Czechoslovakian Academy of Science for which a major duty was to restore its prominence after years of Communist rule.

Ruben provided a testament to Wichterle's primary role as the inventor of the hydrophilic lens in 1980 at the first symposium in London which he attended.

We owe much to Professor Wichterle. He developed the soft lens material. He told me he had started medical training, which unfortunately was stopped by the Nazi invasion of Czechoslovakia. Otherwise he would have been a doctor—a good general practitioner in a practice somewhere—and we would not have had a soft lens. He has become an expert polymer chemist, of course, and he has produced a substance which is still use some 20-odd years after he invented it. He even went a stage further and produced the machinery and method of making a lens, just like Henry Ford did. There is really one big difference: Henry Ford became a millionaire and Professor Wichterle is penniless. The world appreciates the step forward we have made because it has encouraged not only soft lenses, but hard lens research.

Shortly after the departure of the Soviet Union from Czechoslovakia, the US Public Broadcasting System interviewed three Czechs including Wichterle who were identified as entrepreneurs in the repressive system. Wichterle was distinguished for having brought much money to the government, but they also identified him as "the richest man in Czechoslovakia." The one example they used was that Wichterle had one his property the only private tennis court in Prague.

Emergence of hydrophilic lens manufacturers

Bausch & Lomb received substantial rights in 1966 when they sublicensed the Wichterle patent from National Patent Development Corporation. Bausch & Lomb had received the non-exclusive rights to distribute hydrogel lenses based upon Wichterle's technology, but they received exclusive, worldwide rights of the spin casting process. The spin casting process was developed first, and was created because of the non-machinability of the hydrophilic material before or after it had been hydrated. Also, the lenses were very thin and had smooth surfaces. Only after a long and painstaking process, Wichterle developed xerogel lens material which was capable of being polymerized and then modified by a lathe process. It was the non-exclusive license that various companies received throughout the world from National Patent Development Corp, and also allowed the worldwide distribution and eventually provided competition to Bausch & Lomb.

In the United States a profound influence to development occurred when in 1968 the Food and Drug Administration decided to regulate the new hydrophilic material as a drug. Initially, Bausch & Lomb had not expected this, but early reports describing the hydrophilic property as a sponge suitable for bacterial or toxic absorption could possibly be a dangerous product. At the time, there was no FDA device regulation, and the soft lens was defined as a drug, providing a unique challenge to both FDA and B&L. Certain drug standards were of little or no relevance to a soft lens, but they had to be addressed. An example was there was a pregnancy exclusion for taking a drug (or being fitted with soft lens) unless the appropriate testing had been done, so the initial FDA approval in 1971 had a pregnancy exclusion. A second example was in the mid 1970's B&L wanted to develop a lens for presbyopic correction which caused a long period of frustration. The FDA considered this a new indication, of no bearing to the initial hyeropia or myopia usage. However, the FDA had no regulations by which they might evaluate the optical characteristics of the lenses.

In the United States, Bausch & Lomb had the lead on FDA testing due to its early position, and it commenced marketing in 1971. International distribution in Europe actually somewhat earlier, but because of the exigencies of FDA approval, the next company, Warner Lambert (now Ciba Vision) did not receive approval of the Bionite material until 26 months later.

The most prominent international competitor to Bausch & Lomb was National Patent Development Company(NPDC) who in addition to receiving the original worldwide license through the Czechoslovakian government, started companies in various countries for the lathing of the hydrogel.

Three countries outside the United States contributed greatly to soft lens development. The first was Australia which represented a microcosm for soft lens development. Hydron supplied the materials and knowhow to some of the previous hard lens laboratories, but these already had a capability to start and to progress with the new soft lens. Australian optometrists who were the primary fitters also were sophisticated contact lens practitioners who evaluated and presented feedback on new developments in the highly personalized market. Toric soft lenses and thinner hydrogel lenses were products of lathe cut methods and found to have favorable properties. In addition, the small market supported the development of the Corneal & Contact Lens Research Unit of the University of New South Wales, along with other college contact lens units where individual optometrists contributed 50 cents to a research fund collected by contact lens laboratories and distributed to the three optometry schools.

England was a sophisticated market which practitioners more slowly changed from hard lenses to soft, but research and development of successful companies as well as astute researchers in both optometry and ophthalmology led to significant developments. As early as 1970, two companies modified the formulation of polyhema and produced high water content lenses that were thought to sustain continuous lens wear. They were John DeCarle and the

Cooper Permalens(Cooper Labs), and Philip Cordrey with the Sauflon contact lens (Contact Lens Mfr Ltd).

Germany is distinctive for having taken its precise manufacturing techniques for hard lenses and applying them to soft lenses. Companies such as Titmus Weicon and Wohlk produced very good lenses which performed well and were accepted, but they were slow in determining what parameters were essential to a flexible soft lens.

The US, European, and Australian markets suggested the benefits that could be attained from the independently developed technologies. Bausch & Lomb spanning most markets produced what might today be considered a superior, physiological lens at the time with its thinness and smooth surface finish. In most major countries except Germany, B&L was a major force. They were also cognizant of the microbiological and toxicological issues that were expected by the approvals of contact lenses as well as from solution manufacturers such as Alcon, Allergan, and Barnes Hinds. Solution manufacturers had international distribution and benefitted from the extensive testing required for FDA.

A negative aspect of Bausch & Lomb Soflens contact lenses was the series design having the same anterior surface curves, but with aspherical posterior curvatures that complicated fitting and optical effects. The US also had the FDA influence which would eventually be important to the international order leading to physiological and microbiological improvements. Australia had a sophisticated practitioner base which developed order to an infinite variety of lens specifications. While theoretically every lens parameter was available, they produced quality lenses that were tested and optimized by practitioner experience and the optometry schools. In the UK, the de Carle and Sauflon lenses provided a fruitful set of new materials from which extended lens wear and the potential in higher oxygen-permeable lenses would become known.

Through the 1970's spin cast and lathe-cut lens options produced an interesting research dichotomy which became part of the need for interaction between researchers from the United States and the rest of the world. Also, gas permeable hard lenses of different materials became available with advantages, but also some significant problems compared to the PMMA lenses. There were a myriad of contact lens solutions and disinfection techniques that developed, flourished, and occasionally disappeared as the standards of one country were applied to other countries. Chlorohexidine-based solutions were causing allergic effects, even after they survived US FDA approval. Some lenses were capable of being heat disinfected, but further problems developed from surface and bulk lens deposition.

Chapter 2

Response to Challenges of the Expansive Contact Lens Field

Forces Leading to a Contact Lens Association

The enlargement of the soft contact lens field began the emergence of international and national corporations. The newness and expansiveness of the field led to different emphases around the world.

A self appointed Steering Committee was formed to explore the concept of an International Contact Lens Association. The committee consisted of Montague Ruben, Raymond Myers, Brien Holden, Miguel Refojo, Robert Koetting, and Antonio Gassett. Myers, in his international position at a traditionally US firm (Bausch & Lomb), had a perspective of the international disparities and explored the concept of an association for 12-18 months before the committee met. Brien Holden was emerging in his international role by traveling between Australia, the US, and Europe. Both were formulating the strengths and the deficiencies of informational flow and responses by the manufacturers. Montague Ruben represented a forward thinking researcher, author, and ophthalmologist, and he had many connections throughout the world. Robert Koetting from St. Louis was well known in America and internationally by his large clinical practice, the clinical research from large populations, and his influence within professional circles. Antonio Gassett, MD was a young researcher from Gainesville, Florida whose interests were strong with contact lens research and was seemingly making significant strides. Josh Josephson recalls as an invited attendee in 1970-71, "I was a guest speaker at the first ever soft contact lens symposium held in Gainesville, Florida, organized by Herb Kaufman and Tony Gassett."

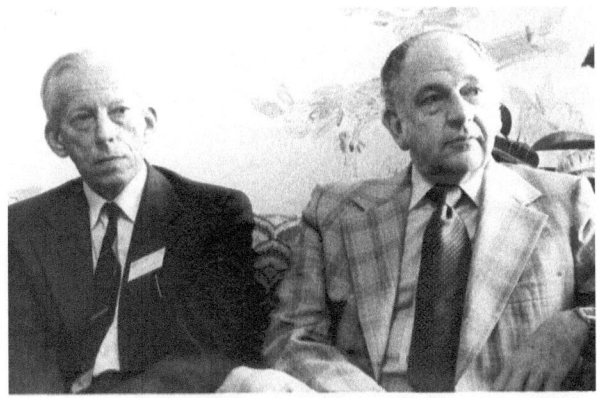

Robert Koetting, Co-founder with ISCLR Patron Otto Wichterle

For a period of 3-6 months, the founding group discussed how the professions might expand and integrate contact lens research and disseminate such information. Manufacturers were making great efforts to get ophthalmologists to fit the contact lenses, as well as optometrists. The potential of contact lenses economically, in many countries with a national health care system, as well as their therapeutic and drug release use, stimulated many ophthalmologists. Also, ophthalmology and their expertise were an important component to the challenges that were obvious in contact lens research.

Yet, bringing together ophthalmology and optometry was always difficult let alone doing this on a worldwide level. In the organizations of optometry and ophthalmology, there was little contact between the groups, although many ophthalmologists and optometrists had friendly relations. The potential for a successful effort internationally lay in avoiding domestic(national) quarrels while exchanging information of mutual value.

Montague Ruben

Montague Ruben possessed the international reputation in 1978 around which an international contact lens organization could most likely develop. Ruben's early background before ophthalmology was as an optometrist(ophthalmic optician). Further information on Ruben is in Appendix 10. Because of his chief position as Consultant Ophthalmologist and Director of the Contact Lenses and Prosthetics at Moorfields Eye Hospital, he held a position in medical contact lenses that was unique to the rest of the world. At the time Moorfields Eye Hospital was one of several eye hospitals in London, and was also the referral eye hospital for a 12 other eye hospitals where much of the secondary and tertiary eye care occurred in the British Health Care System. The department he ran consisted of several ophthalmologists, 4-6 optometrists, at least 10 contact lens fitters and technical personnel, and a specialized hard and soft contact laboratory. At least 2 contact lens opticians spent full time in doing scleral PMMA fittings, and there was a Pediatric Clinic once a week which kept aphakic neonates and infants wearing their continuous wear lenses.

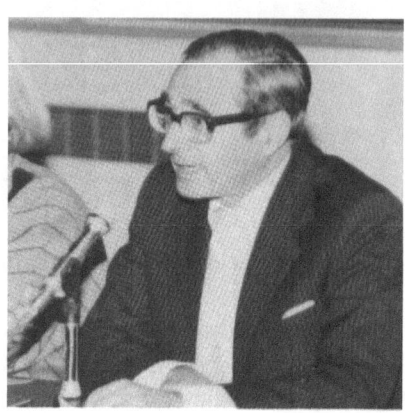

Montague Ruben; Co-founder(1984)

Numerous research projects were occurring at Moorfields Eye Hospital which he and others published. Ruben's academic affiliations were at the Institute of Ophthalmology and City University in London. Michel Guillon chose Ruben as his advisor, and he spent his pre-registration year, as well as subsequent years at Moorfields. Other ISCLR charter members worked with and collaborated with Ruben. Nur Ahmed, David Lobascher, Judith Morris, Geoffrey Woodward, Ray Myers, and later Roger Buckley as Ruben's successor were all Moorfields alumni.

The UK was closest to a model of what contact lens practice might be as envisioned in organizations where optometry and ophthalmology coexisted and learned from each other. The British Contact Lens Association included many ophthalmologists as members as well as optometry. The Medical Contact Lens Association did exist separately, but typically the optometrists practicing in the hospitals participated as non-members in their specialized organization.

Monty Ruben worked with Harold Ridley in his earlier years at Moorfields. Ridley had conceived and developed the first intraocular implants and also used scleral contact lenses. When word spread that Wichterle had invented the soft lens material, Wichterle visited Moorfields with NPDC one afternoon in 1963 and met with Ridley and a young ophthalmologist named Montague Ruben. Wichterle recounts this in his book, *Reflections,* that he was impressed with the young Ruben with whom he developed a close relationship. Ruben and Wichterle collaborated as much as possible given the restrictions of his country's Communist regime.

Ruben also spoke among ophthalmological and optometric groups in Europe, the United States as well as Japan and enjoyed a number of positions as speaker and author of numerous papers on contact lenses and related topics, and as honorary chairman and moderator. When Myers was at Moorfields for his one year research fellowship, he had an almost continuous flow of optometric and ophthalmological observers from numerous countries throughout the world, who flowed through the Hospital as a prime means of advanced education. Ruben's knowledge of the world contact lens order, particularly in ophthalmology, would be instrumental in organizing international efforts to develop an International organization.

In the early 1980's Ruben had been at Moorfields Eye Hospital for many years, and he and his wife Margaret decided to come to the United States for as much as five years instead of remaining at Moorfields until his retirement. He chose to look at various American optometry schools and was impressed by the efforts at the University of Houston College of Optometry to establish a contact lens institute. Among the individuals he knew he would work were Council member Jan Bergmanson and Irvin Borish.

When Ruben returned to the states several years later, he would retire. He informed the ISCLR Executive Council that he would no longer remain involved in research and his professional pursuits, but would retire to Broadstairs, Kent and his Spanish home near S'Agaro. After his last meeting in 1986, Ruben remained interested in ISCLR pursuits in perennial reports by Michel Guillon and Ray Myers.

Brien Holden

Brien Holden was a lecturer at the University of New South Wales in Sydney, Australia, when he began to travel extensively with a message of the state of contact lenses in Australia. He had graduated from the University of Melbourne, and later became a Ph.D. candidate at City University in London in the 1960's. In 1973, Holden visited the US where he first met Raymond Myers at Bausch & Lomb in Rochester, New York. Myers arranged a tour of Bausch & Lomb which included meetings with various officials. Holden had a characteristic brutal honesty which was slightly less refined compared to today. He proceeded to tell B&L what was wrong with their lenses, and more unbelievably, talked about products readily available in the Australian marketplace that were still on the drawing board at B&L. Of significant importance was the growing realization that B&L lenses performed poorly with vision which could be contrasted in Australia, where sophisticated practitioners were achieving excellent results with the availability of a variety of lenses. Holden left creating a disturbance from executives who disbelieved his assessment and the Australian results.

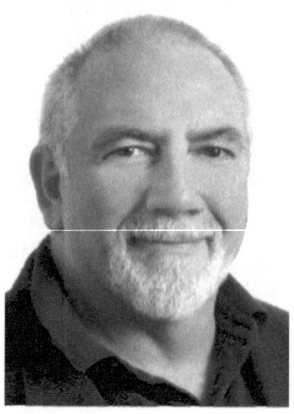

Brien Holden; Co-Founder

The next year Holden was to return this time to the American Academy of Optometry, and would visit Rochester immediately after the meeting. Myers' job before he left for meeting was to arrange meetings with executives. Meetings that Myers arranged could be classified into various levels depending upon the input or influence of the professional visitor: one level might include a tour with some discussions and the highest level was for those having substantial input and included some executives. Holden's first visit was a second level visit, but it was clear for the next year that executives felt he should be accorded the lowest level.

However, at the Academy meeting, Holden who was accompanied by Keith Masnick jointly reported on the status of Australian contact lenses as well as the performance of toric soft contact lenses. (Holden BA., 51(10):1974: 743-9) Toric lenses had barely been considered because they were not prominent elsewhere in the world and Bausch & Lomb had constraints from their manufacturing method. When Myers and Holden arrived in Rochester, the tour changed considerably to the highest lever with the B&L Soflens President and vice presidents starting the morning in a joint scientific conference.

Holden and other Australian leaders had developed a funding resource through a voluntary assessment by optometrists paid through the laboratories and be distributed to the universities for contact lens research. Holden expanded his international influence and his preeminence in the contact lens field. He confronted the dramatic differences in knowledge as well as in practice. Soft lenses were being fitted outside the US by individuals not having the physiological and a microbiological background now included in the hydrogel literature. He as well as Myers became aware that dissemination of knowledge required specific education for clinicians, building from the level they were trained.

More than any other founder, Holden traveled the world with its great contact lens diversity, from countries to manufacturers, and initially disseminated the Association and Society plan internationally. Holden can be attributed as having suggested and defended the need of a research society, as well as contributing extensively throughout its 30 year history. Past President and chemist Miguel Refojo has proposed, "If the ISCLR named Wichterle as Patron in honor of his contribution to the contact lens field, then they should name Brien Holden the 'Godfather.' This is not only for his contributions to the development of the contact lens field, but particularly for his leadership and influence in ISCLR affairs."

Raymond I. Myers

Raymond Myers entered optometry school in 1966 at Indiana University having graduated from the University of Notre Dame. At Notre Dame, he became very involved in student organizations, and in optometry school he became a co-founder of the American Optometric Student Association. He continued with an interest in association activity as the Director of Career Guidance for the American Optometric Association after he graduated from optometry from Indiana University. In 1972, Myers along with other AOA officials sat across from William Coombs, Executive Vice President of Bausch & Lomb Soflens Division. Coombs was trying to rescue Bausch & Lomb from a devastating but financially successful introduction and Myers' interest was piqued by the potential of the field. Myers returned to his contact lens interests which had been nurtured by his mentor Irvin Borish, while at Indiana University. Myers accepted a position as Bausch & Lomb manager of international professional services and external research activity in 1973.

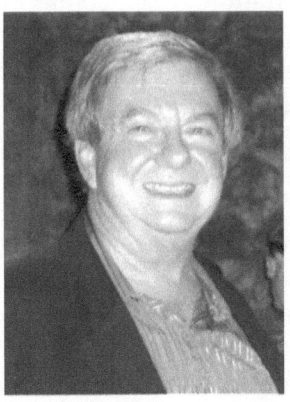

Raymond Myers; Co-Founder

Myers' international professional service position was initially incongruous at Bausch & Lomb which was largely a successful American company with a US contact lens monopoly, but the international marketplace highlighted the significant advantages and the weaknesses of the Bausch & Lomb Soflens Contact Lens. American practitioners as well B&L management did not recognize the variety in lens offerings considering the spin cast soft lenses with limited parameters were the only options available. Additionally, the research challenges of the US were diverted toward microbiological directions by virtue of FDA's approval as a drug. In the five years with B&L Myers, Holden and Ruben's paths crossed frequently. In 1977 Myers resigned from Bausch & Lomb to begin a research fellowship at Moorfields Eye Hospital.

Myers has often been involved in the creation and establishment of new organizations and sometimes new concepts or directions. In addition to his college organizational development, professional services and relations was new to the ophthalmic field and required a more sophisticated form of practitioner education and interaction than the more sedate ophthalmic industry before it. Later, Myers established at the University of Missouri-St. Louis the Materials Science and Chemistry Symposium on Contact Lenses after ISCLR development. He saw the need primarily for the chemistry oriented people in industry and academia to develop cooperative efforts toward the next generation of contact lens materials. Since 1996, Myers' interests have been toward laser lens modification of the crystalline lens for presbyopia and other conditions which has incorporated a new direction largely defined by his intellectual property.

Holden summarized Myers' role at the close of the 1st Symposium in London as well as subsequent times. "Myers was the original instigator of this Society back when he worked with Bausch and Lomb. He wanted to set up an international association to assist communication between societies. That ideal went by the political wayside, but out of that was born the idea of a research meeting of some scientists to discuss issues in which we had an interest."

Michel Guillon

Michel Guillon fortuitously began his tenure with ISCLR as Montague Ruben's graduate student and attended as the recorder of the Steering Committee meeting in June, 1978. He received his PhD from City University in London and proceeded to start his own research institute, OTG Research and Consulting, where he has conducted research in contact lens optics, dry eyes, tear film, sports vision, and refractive surgery. He was also the co-editor with Montague Ruben on his book Contact Lens Practice in 1998 (Ruben &

Guillon, Contact Lens Practice, 1994) and an author of 11 chapters in various textbooks.

Guillon has been a tireless and active contributor first as the Secretary of the Society and the assistant program chair for the first meeting. In 1999 ISCLR president Guillon had substantial roles in program development and implementation through the early years of the Symposia. He was also involved with Kenneth Polse in editing the transcripts of the first four Symposia. The first proceedings were monumental starting with the transcriptions which were often done by the society and without the professional sound recording methods. Although Past President Kenneth Polse was primarily responsible, the efforts were often a result of the two setting down for as long as a week and interpreting the wide range of topics and language accents. A variety of ISCLR officers including Guillon gauged the effectiveness of the sessions of the early programs to enhance interaction and discussion that was first based upon the designated panel and secondarily on the input from the rest of the attendees. Between the outward controls of time or slide limits were also indoctrination and gentle nudging which many moderators learned through the controls of Guillon and Holden. These would include modifications between sessions to the meeting format or room design.

Guillon, Myers, and Holden were interacting constantly to all of the meetings between 1980 and at least 1995 in the meeting arrangements, membership, financial matters, and program implementation. There was even travel among their respective locales, both for ISCLR reasons and collaborations. Guillon spent approximately one year in Sydney. For this reason, their relationship was always close, mostly cordial, but was often intense particularly in several days of planning before the actual meeting. Consequently, there were many tales of interaction that are important to the society because the three created a continuity and base with the Executive Council contributing most of the direction and the changing officers of President, President-Elect and Program Chairman inserting the new ideas.

Robert A. Koetting

Robert Koetting is a clinical optometrist from St. Louis, Missouri who maintained a practice limited to contact lenses for 25 years until 1986. A limited contact lens practice without any vestige of eyeglasses was practically unknown outside of St. Louis, and it was in part a result of a relationship between optometry and ophthalmology. Prior to the advent of contact lens institutes and multi-center studies, Koetting reported observational studies with large patient populations drawing certain conclusions which came from a large, limited contact lens practice. He was both a favored speaker and author in various journals, and was an early diplomate and chairperson in the American

Academy of Optometry, and founder and chair of the American Optometric Association Contact Lens Section.

At the time of ISCLR's founding Koetting was traveling frequently outside the United States and was cognizant of the dichotomies in international practice. He was also capable of leading American optometry in a direction of the "International Contact Lens Association."

Chapter 3

The Early ISCLR

A New International Contact Lens Association

The conditions existing in hydrogel development throughout the world demonstrated the opportunity to advance the field by communication and interaction of the different regions. On June 24-25, 1978, the Steering Committee for the proposed International Contact Lens Association (ICLA) met in London at the Royal College of Surgeons. The original plan was to form an international association with ophthalmology and optometry. The effort was complicated because there were different patterns of fitting among ophthalmologists in the various countries. Also, optometry was not uniformly defined as a profession or present in the various countries. The degree to which hydrogels were being accepted in most countries, however, was leading to both optometry and ophthalmology participating in contact lens fitting. Heretofore, hard contact lenses were a technical arena, albeit one with medical indications, where very few ophthalmologists chose to be involved except through opticians and technicians. Further, continuing education and international coordination could have a favorable effect upon interprofessional relationships especially if there was an organization which incorporated ophthalmology and optometry.

One possible structure for the Association was to establish an "organization of organizations" by bringing together national contact lens organizations(Contact Lens Association of Ophthalmology(US), British Contact Lens Association, and the Australian Contact Lens Society). There were not many organizations dedicated to contact lenses in the various countries although there may have been broad based associations with contact lens sections. In fact, an international organization might stimulate this. No country, with the exception of the UK and Scandinavian countries, had multi-professional contact lens organizations.

Another structure would be to make the individual as the member rather than the national organization. They would be optometrists and ophthalmologists and researchers who would enter the ICLA directly. The Steering Committee had worked out where national organizations and individuals could become members, with a substantial effort to stimulate further national organizations.

The initial organizers or Steering Committee consisted of Montague Ruben, Raymond Myers, Brien Holden, Robert Koetting, and Antonio Gassett. Previously, each had selected a number of acquaintances for the purpose of establishing this new organization. Each wrote a letter to their colleagues stressing several issues: first, the considerable disparity of contact lens knowledge internationally which needed to be narrowed. Second, the hydrogel explosion resulted in unique contributions from different countries where past contributions and a new coalition would likely result in an international information exchange. Third, the international effort would combine the efforts of the two professions which were of considerable importance to the future development of the field.

The preponderance of responses from invited professionals was favorable, and the need for this organization was clear. Tabulated responses from respondents were as follows: solicitations by Ruben, Holden, Myers, and Koetting numbered 24 Yes; 1 No, and 6 no responses. The plan then was for the organizers to meet in London and establish the new International Contact Lens Association. Myers was already with Ruben in London at Moorfields Eye Hospital for a one year fellowship, and Holden would come for one month on a sabbatical visit during Myers' visit. This meant that only Koetting and Gassett would fly to London from St. Louis and Gainesville, respectively. The group received financial support from International Hydron Corp., with successful subsidiaries including the UK and Europe, Australia, and the US.

The constitutional meeting occurred at the Boardroom of the Moorfields Eye Hospital and began at 9 a.m. on Saturday, June 24-25, 1978. Antonio Gassett cancelled the trip at the last minute having run into some local political heat but it was never understood whether this was for political or personal reasons. Holden was to arrive about two hours late in the morning, because of a late flight from Helsinki, Finland. Fortuitously, Ruben had asked that Michel Guillon, his graduate student and Moorfields intern, be the scribe for the group.

While waiting for Holden to arrive, Ruben, Koetting, Myers, and Guillon spent most of this time discussing the first major issue—how to organize the ICLA considering the organizational and political realities in the Europe and United States. No problem appeared to be intractable, but the issues were complicated and required extended discussion.

Ruben was the key to the analysis because he was interpreting the acceptance of responders from his own extensive personal relationships, the absence of responses from certain people, and the others to whom he had spoken. Despite Gassett's non-appearance, the US ophthalmologists and optometrists appeared to support in principle the concept as was seen in the numbers of letters. The impediments appeared most to be ophthalmologists in Europe where the variances in educational backgrounds among optometrists of different countries made this a difficult union. Opinion molders would cause difficulties in acceptance. Possibly the most significant example was Jules Francoise, the dean of European ophthalmology from the University of Ghent in Belgium. Francoise's influence in European ophthalmology was unparalleled at the time. Also, a few years before the ISCLR was conceived when Myers was the International Professional Services Manager for Bausch & Lomb, he welcomed hundreds of professionals in Rochester. During Francoise's visit Myers was instructed to refrain from any involvement because of Francoise's known opposition to optometry.

Despite these difficulties, Ruben and Myers believed that an array of fortunate circumstances would reduce interprofessional rivalries and result in communication and research interactions at least in the proposed association. Also, the Committee felt that interprofessional relationships nationally would lead to national contact lens associations perhaps with the same interprofessional model.

When Holden arrived several hours late, he showed obvious complications with a late flight. However, he summarized his previous day's activity which was on the yacht of Antii Vannas who later became an ISCLR officer, collaborator and friend of Holden. The previous day was a long and festive trip into the evening and everything that followed on Holden's trip was fatiguing.

Upon Holden's arrival, the committee summarized the problems as well as the likely solutions, although by then the direction had not been completely determined. The summary was shorten when Holden who seemed somewhat impatient to learn of the interprofessional problems. Holden posed the question, "Why are we trying to establish this organization?" Without doubt, it was to bring about an active exchange of information and speed up future developments. "So why not avoid all the political problems," Holden exclaimed, "and establish a research society of active researchers within academia, ophthalmology, and optometry?"

Myers and Ruben initially resisted this approach because the Association was possible considering the initial favorable, but problematic analysis. The more the Steering Committee deliberated they agreed it was the dissemination of research, rather than the collegiality of a larger group, that would make the difference in contact lens research and development. The group decided on the Research Society concept and quickly settled on the name, the International Society for Contact Lens Research.

Pre-First Symposium Planning

A significant problem became apparent because many of the initially people contacted had a political leaning, rather than a solid research background that was needed for a research organization. Ruben suggested that he write back to all indicating the new direction of a Research Society as well as acknowledging our thanks of their individual support for the original concept. The Board proceeded later to contact a new group of potential members, some who were on the original list. A problem ensued because some individuals who were not invited again were clearly miffed. But the organizing committee was intent on ensuring that the credentials of prospective members reflected the highest level of research, without making this group unduly academic.

The greatest obstacle was in defining clinical research which was an important part of the discussion and deliberations for a future meeting. Starting with the inaugural meeting, a standard for the clinical members was defined which would include a history of publications and some originality in contact lens research based upon publication in refereed journals. The inclusion of non-academics, albeit original contributors of the caliber of future Ruben medalist Donald Korb was therefore expected and welcomed. The problem came with individuals who were part of the political contact lens establishment and whose research was not original or current.

Among the researchers, there was recognition of the role of ophthalmologists who in some incidences were contact lens researchers but were less likely to perform directly the role as contact lens practitioners. But the medical role of contact lenses and potential complications being discussed in the United States made this a crucial group to gain participation.

Manufacturers' role in the organization was thought to be crucial, because in the growing hydrophilic international manufacturing field, a relatively few companies were emerging as the forces behind development. Myers & Holden were particularly aware of the strengths within the companies. Although companies were emerging with professional panels and consultants in the broad areas of development and marketing, ISCLR offered something which no one manufacturer could duplicate, which was an independent "think tank" that provided direction to basic and clinical research broadly enough for the membership as well as the individual manufacturers. The early ISCLR organizers felt it was necessary to retain independence from manufacturers, but still gain their input and participation.

The financial strain that a new international organization had on its members became an important issue. A significant number of academics would find the added costs to be a challenge, and some offset of international travel costs was needed. Associating this meeting with another conference was considered possible, but the meetings were either themselves very lengthy or the meetings directed toward only one eye care professional. Manufacturers would then be invited to participate, make a financial contribution, and be able to have a limited number of attendees which would likely be from the corporations' research and development staffs.

The last element of manufacturer participation was how to recognize corporate researchers and input. Staff researchers could apply to the ISCLR using the same standards that were set for other basic and clinical researchers in contact lenses and related areas.

The New Research Society

Shortly after the inaugural meeting a Steering Committee for the new Society was formed consisting of Montague Ruben, Brien Holden, Raymond Myers, and David Miller. Miller was an ophthalmologist and associate professor with Harvard University, suggested at the first meeting and was invited due to his initial interest in the gaining acceptance by American ophthalmology of a limited research society. Ruben and Myers were responsible for much of the communication that contacted potentially new members, starting with the potential list that Steering Committee members developed. Ruben was also crucial in building European participation among ophthalmologists and contact lens researchers in Europe where limited support was displayed for the original "international contact lens association." The presence of European ophthalmological researchers of the caliber of M Kraznov(Russia), H W Roth(Germany), Peter Wright(England), and Baronet(France), along with Hikaru Hamano(Japan) established an interprofessional foundation in the early stages.

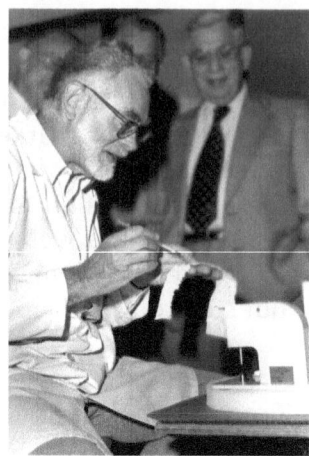

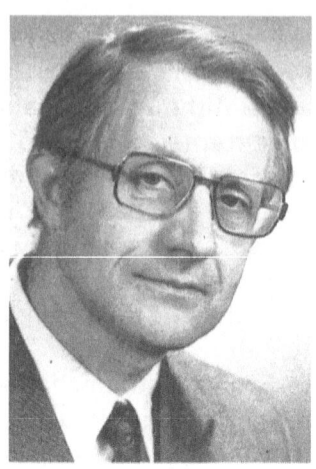

Irving Fatt was a staunch representative of the power of science and the infallibility of scientific principles

Guenter Forst was an early and consistent Symposium attendee who was both a Councillor and moderator

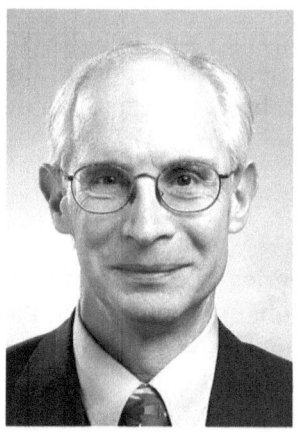

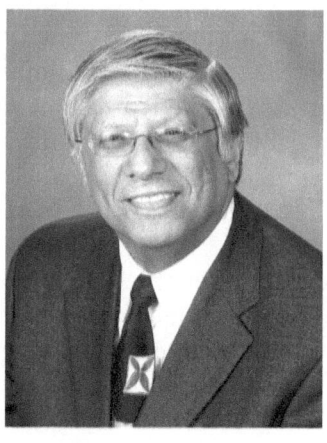

Michael Harris became ISCLR's de facto legal counsel

Nizar Hirji was an active member and researcher after which his distinguished career was in UK professional and continuing education endeavors

Myers and Ruben communicated frequently starting with a list of 25 who were favorably responsive in the first Steering Committee meeting. Holden was spreading the word in his travels. Letters went out to another group of prospective members and further included personal contact, especially to those who were not originally contacted.

Among American ophthalmologists, the idea of a limited contact lens research society was attractive to some invitees, but opposition from others who were not invited placed considerable pressure. A relatively few applied for membership, especially in the first round of 1978-79. It would eventually take individuals starting with Michael Lemp and Perry Binder to define and reduce opposition of the ISCLR.

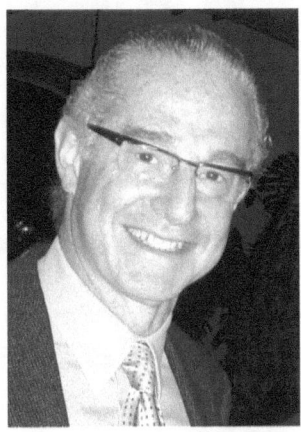 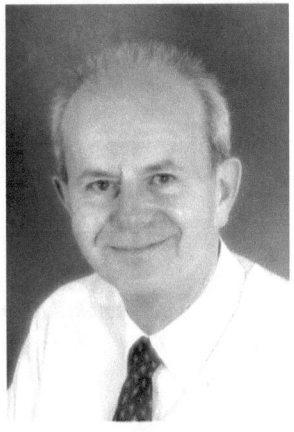

Joshua Josephson initially represented a skilled Canadian clinician having broader contact lens availability than American clinicians

As a successor to Ruben at Moorfields Eye Hospital, Roger Buckley was active and an ISCLR Vice President

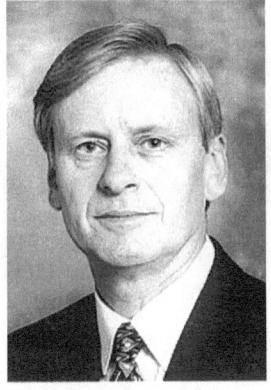 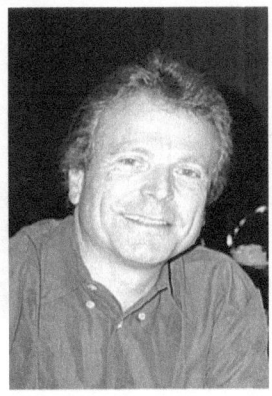

Jonathon Kersley brought about greater ISCLR acceptance in the European ophthalmological community

Peter Fanti as a German Augenoptiker, leader, and editor, has attended all Symposia

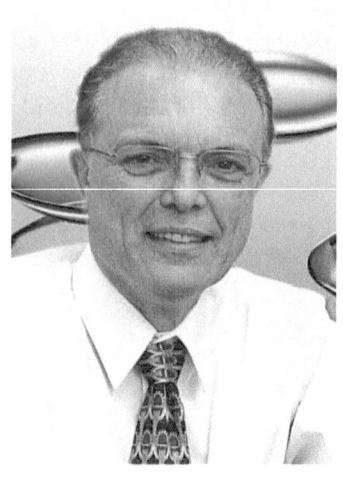

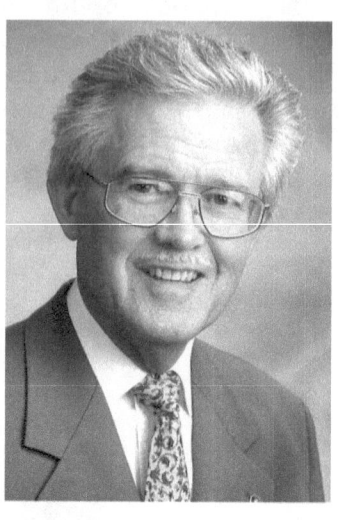

Anthony Philips, renown book author, was in the UK at the ISCLR inception and moved to Adelaide, Australia

Sven Nielson consistently reported on a wide variety of medical issues with contact lens wear

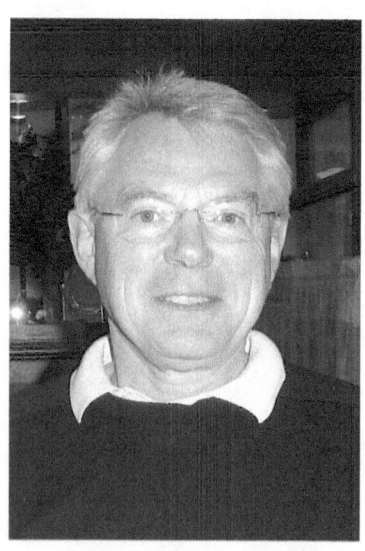

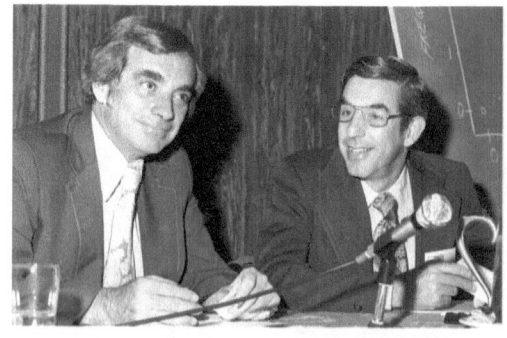

Michael Port is one of the original British researchers to become an ISCLR member

Morton Sarver and Maurice Poster were prolific clinical researchers with PMMA and proceeded to make great contributions with hydrophilic lenses

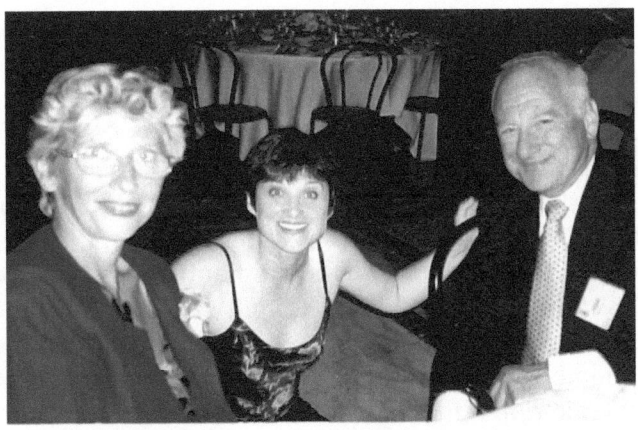

Pierre and Brigitte Rocher with Barbara Caffery

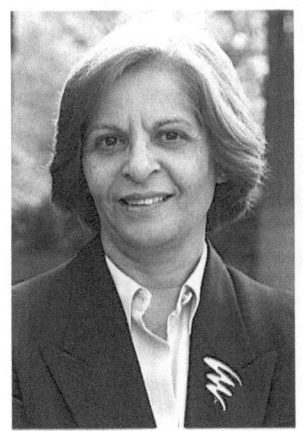

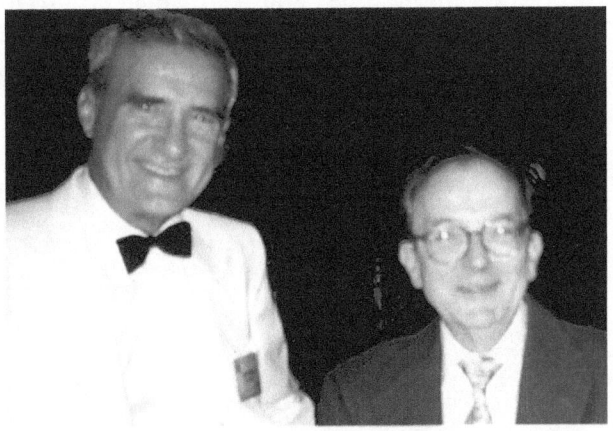

Sarita Soni reported on a wide number of clinical lens applications

Long time Friends Tony Henriquez and Donald Korb. Henriquez made local arrangements for the 1986 S'Agaro symposium

From the beginning it was clear that periodic meetings were the crucial function for the organization, but probably not the only role that ISCLR would have. Planning for the first meeting began one year earlier at meetings at Association for Research in Vision and Ophthalmology and the American Academy of Optometry.

At the 1980 London Symposium, the Council originally appointed by the Steering Committee held a lengthy meeting on the future format knowing that certain exigencies explained below required a different format for the inaugural, London Symposium. Future meetings, however, would incorporate the design that was hotly discussed by the Council. Holden, Fatt, Lemp, and Polse were among the active contributors. The Council assessed the different meetings they attended and what would come from them. It was clear at this time that ISCLR membership would be limited, that publicity and publication from this meeting would be limited, and that the most important outcome would be from group discussion rather than formal papers. Current meeting styles of the Academies of optometry and ophthalmology and the Association for Research in Vision and Ophthalmology(ARVO) emphasized individual attainment, with a relatively small time spent for discussion. Panel discussions at typical meetings had interaction, but often did not necessarily generate forward thinking.

The concept "think tank" came early. Irvin Fatt and Kenneth Polse were familiar with meetings like the Gordon Conferences which were held often in rustic and remote areas and were small groups interacting on limited topics with maximum deliberations. However, this was not completely what the ISCLR would need, and summarizing the future, it would take upwards to 10 years to perfect a format that characterizes the current ISCLR meetings.

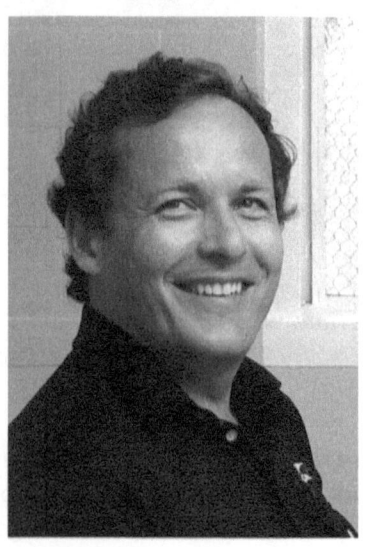

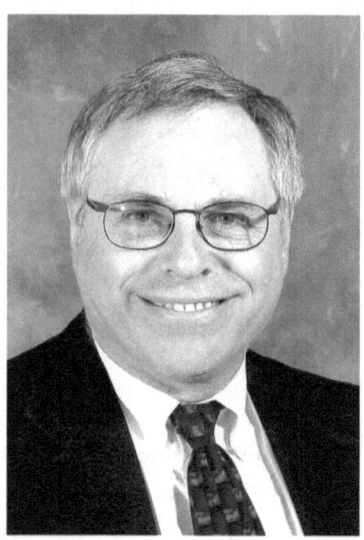

Aanti Vannas was a staunch ISCLR supporter and its interprofessional nature until his death in 2006

Barry Weissman has provided a broad perspective in research based upon his medical contact lens practice

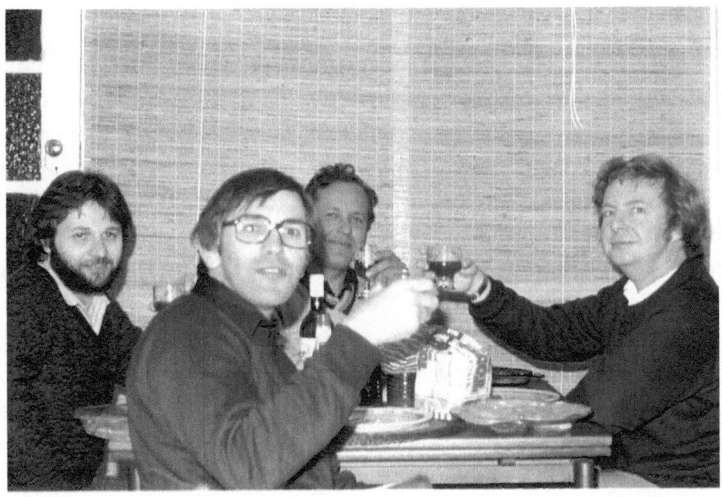

The meeting discussion continues into the night among MIchel Guillon, Richard Pearson, Aanti Vannas, and Raymond Myers

First Symposium—London, England—September 5-6, 1980

London was a centralized site for the first meeting and was appropriate considering its origin from the first Steering Committee meeting. Also, membership numbers from the UK, next to the US, were the largest. The attendance of 50 included about ½ non-members. London was also a central site for Europe and UK's reasonably good relationship between ophthalmology and optometry definitely jumpstarted the reputation of a multiprofessional meeting.

Ruben succinctly summarized the first meeting and the history and intent of the ISCLR in opening remarks to the gathering.

> *It is my pleasant duty to welcome you to London, to this meeting, and to this beautiful hall which the Royal College of Surgeons has been kind enough to let us use. The International Society for Contact Lens Research is now in being and we are pleased to announce that the patron of this new research society will be Professor Otto Wichterle. This Society was created out of a failed conception: the original plan was to have an International Council for Contact Lens Societies which combined all the professions in a single interest. We are not ready for that at this time, but certainly some of you may see it in your lifetimes. This Research Society wishes to avoid any political considerations*

and is concerned only with research in contact lens practice and the allied sciences. Your membership in this Society is recognition of your contributions to contact lens research, with the emphasis on research. I realize that there are many non-members present at this first meeting and I hope that you eventually will have the necessary qualifications for membership in this Society. Some future meetings may be limited to members only and we may have open congresses from time to time. The total number of members will be severely limited: therefore, those people who are elected to membership must consider it a distinction. There are, unfortunately, a few ophthalmologists who are not here today because certain problems prevent them from following their own consciences. It is sad that meetings such as this that deal only with science are subject to such political influences. It is even sadder to know that such eminent ophthalmologists, practicing in countries we assume to have the greatest democracies in the world are working under such shadows.

The first slate of officers consisted of the following group:

- Patron: Otto Wichterle
- President: Montague Ruben
- President Elect: Brien Holden
- Vice President: Richard Hill
- Vice President: Michael Lemp
- Vice President: Miguel Refojo
- Secretary-Treasurer: Raymond Myers
- Assistant Secretary: Michel Guillon

Original Council members in addition to the officers were Leo Carney, Wulf Ehrich, Irving Fatt, Hikaru Hamano, Frank Holly, Richard Keates, Robert Koetting, Donald Korb, Michail Krasnov, John Larke, Gerald Lowther, Ian Mackie, Robert Mandell, David Maurice, Saiichi Mishima, Kenneth Polse, Maurice Poster, Hans-Walter Roth, Janet Stone, Paul White, and Peter Wright.

Original manufacturers and financial sponsors were Allergan, Alcon Laboratories and Medical, Allergan, Bausch & Lomb, Polymer Technology Corporation, CIBA Vision Corporation, Pilkington, Vistakon, Wesley Jessen, Biocompatibles, and Coopervision. Important scientific contributions from manufacturers in the first Symposium included Stuart Eriksen from Allergan and Kiran Randieri from Alcon.

Also, it was an honor to have ISCLR's patron Otto Wichterle whose participation gave the society its foundation. Montague Ruben and Miguel Refojo had previous multiple encounters with Wichterle.

`The two day Symposium on Friday and Saturday was held at the Royal College of Surgeons in London, a stately and formal site which was to remain the model site for the next two symposia. The meeting hotel was separated by several blocks from the College. The first Symposium chairperson was President-Elect Brien Holden which began the tradition to this day for Presidents-Elect who are elected at the previous meeting. The issues at the time for which there were panels set up included corneal edema and oxygen needs, physiological and pathological responses to contact lenses, systems for disinfection, lens spoliation, and new measurement techniques. The panels consisted of a large number of individuals and the embryonic plan to maximize discussion was hindered by too many topics and panels without control of the speakers. Nevertheless, issues and people would identify themselves as important and unique contributors to future meetings.

Irvin Fatt, an engineer and academician from the University of California, began his contributions with this first meeting in a lively exchange on corneal oxygen needs and measurement techniques, which continued as a major topic in many future symposia. With Holden chairing the session, a controversy began between the advocates of individuals including Fatt where oxygen measurements were strictly based upon physical measurement techniques in comparison to clinically measured techniques.

Frank Holly had a distinguished career in tear analysis which he carried through at many of the first meetings. He and Miguel Refojo distinguished themselves among the transcribers of the proceedings, because their accents became the burden for transcription of their important contributions.

Materials properties were not considered as a major topic in the first symposium, although the challenges of spoliation were a topic in which Wichterle participated. After listening to the nuts and bolts difficulties that were known at the time for soft lenses, Wichterle's prescient comments were as follows:

> Is it worth investing a great deal of research on this problem? There is one solution that would eliminate all the problems of deposition: Once deposits occur, we could reject the lens and take a new one! I believe we are now very close to the development of technology which will cause a dramatic drop in the selling price of lenses. Once you are able to buy a lens for one dollar or less, lens spoilage won't play a role. If a lens is spoiled, it will be cheaper to buy a new lens than to buy expensive solutions and a waste time with cleaning.
>
> I remember 17 years ago, in my first speech about these lenses, I predicted that lenses would soon be sold for less than one dollar. I was wrong, it wasn't that soon.

Seven years later, Vistakon from Jacksonville, Florida, somewhat unexpectedly introduced disposable soft lenses with less expensive packaging. It is likely that Charter Member Sheldon Wechsler from the relatively small company was listening!

An event during an evening informal dinner demonstrated another aspect of Wichterle's character. The restaurant was located a cab-ride away in London which the group did in multiple vehicles. After dinner a group of 6 to 8 started to look for a taxi back to the hotel, but they were a bit difficult to find. Wichterle suggested everyone should all walk back. Coming from the oldest one in the group(Wichterle was then 67), no one said no, although there appeared to be little enthusiasm. As they talked and walked, it was clear who the leader was, because Wichterle was always at the head of the group. His lifelong activity as a tennis player was in part a contributor to his stamina.

Chapter 4

A Maturing ISCLR

The London symposium was as significant in developing the organizational structure and future meeting structure as it was to produce the first scientific meeting. The first Council included six future ISCLR Presidents. A Constitution was reviewed and modified to come up with the specific officers, council, and membership qualifications.

The minimum standards for membership were defined by the numbers of papers the applicant authored or coauthored in recognized contact lens or other journals. Clinicians were welcome and their input would be expected in combination with the more basic and academic research efforts. Membership would be limited to 150(later 100).

In 1990 Past President Michael Lemp would summarize the vision of the Society. "The basic framework of the organization was to bring together, in an informal setting, a limited number of individuals from different disciplines, united by their interest and proven expertise in the field of contact lens research. The meetings were designed as an informal exchange of new ideas and leading edge research methodologies prior to publication in established journals. Indeed, the proceedings of these meetings were not to be citable, nor distributed beyond the attendees at the meeting, thus allowing for a free exchange of yet-unproven hypotheses and preliminary results."

Past President Kenneth Polse identifies how the society can continue with the vitality that has kept ISCLR strong for 30 years. "Finally and perhaps most important is that I continue to be impressed with the time and sincerity so many of the members work to make the society what it is today. Without compensation and very few accolades Society members give of their time to improve the society."

Developing a meeting format

The meeting format was one of the most important functions of the Executive Committee and the Council which began during the first Symposium meeting, but extended during each Scientific session and for the next ten years. Forming a limited membership society was being done in order to distinguish the Society from other organizations including Association for Research in Vision in Ophthalmology, the International Society of Contact Lens Specialists, the Academies of Optometry and Ophthalmology, and the national contact lens societies. All of these which were frequented by large memberships were forums for original papers with some discussion and interaction; but they were larger audiences and unfocused when it came to optimizing interactions among the researchers.

The Society eventually adapted the Gordon Conference, as previously discussed, to a think tank format by having a limited number of topics, with minimal presentation, recognizing the importance of all members to an individual topic while singling out a panel, moderator and keynote speaker. An important ingredient was that each member would have input and/or personal gain in every session. Therefore, full attendance at each session was encouraged by tying in the ISCLR stipend which was predicated upon full meeting attendance. Eventually there was further clarification that this would lead to pro-rating the stipend if a member were to leave.

Various changes were gradually made in the meetings.

- Symposium attendance was limited to members or prospective members, and there were a variety of situations where either prominent contact lens officials in the country of the Symposia or even non-member spouses of members were discouraged from attending.
- The physical setup of the meeting was changed and constantly tweaked to facilitate discussion first by the panelists and then inputting the remarks of the audience. Long introductions and responses were discouraged.
- The Board encouraged and eventually tightened the recommendation that members attend at least one of two successive symposia, or lose membership. The one overriding benefit of Society membership was the biennial Symposium, and a small membership encouraged the retention of those who were active.
- The participation of individual members as panelist was largely determined by the topic selection for that year. Although a miscellaneous area was always included, receiving a stipend to attend was not tied to a presentation or being a panelist. Each member did not necessarily make a presentation at each meeting.

- Maximizing interaction in the panels and minimizing individual presentations were the subjects of many meeting alterations, sometimes resulting in modifications during an actual meeting. They included limiting the number of slides for panelists, instructing the moderators, different room arrangements, and timing devices. Summing up and integrating the different topics became the additional burden on senior members as well as the session moderators who became responsible for ensuring and enumerating the conclusions and directions.

- Keynote presentations have often been summaries of a topic under discussion, but meeting organizers also began looking for outside input to broaden the perspective. When the topic required a broader look at new technologies or techniques, a non-member was most often offered a larger stipend than most members or Council. Historically, many of these individuals eventually became members and their attendance may have had a role in a fruitful association with the contact lens field. See Appendix 7 for a list of keynote speakers including those who were not members at the time they were invited.

The length of the scientific sessions changed significantly from the beginning. The London Symposium(1980) was two days; the Montreal(1982) Symposium went to three days which remained the same in the next four meetings. Yet, there was still the belief that a four day meeting was needed, but the three day meetings had become inordinately demanding considering that many were involved in one or more panels as well as attending each and every session. After the 1984 Cambridge meeting, the Council decided that a possible solution for a less strenuous three day meeting would be to select a tropical environment free from urban distractions and split the morning and afternoon sessions with a long lunch hour where individuals could enjoy the sun and recover. The 1986 S'Agaro, Spain began this precedent which continued until a 5 day meeting was started at the 1993 Hayman Island(Australia). A Wednesday day of rest was then included midway in a Monday-Friday schedule which became the basis of all future meetings. Except for the 1990 Monte Carlo and 1997 Florence Symposia, succeeding meetings have been away from urban communities. Three have included a rustic and mountainous ambiance(Jackson Hole(1995), Sun Valley(2001) and Whistler Mountain(2007).

Manufacturers' Role

Manufacturers have always been crucial ISCLR participants because of their R&D role. Although the contact lens field existed before Wichterle's grand invention, multinational companies have had the most significant influence on developments in successive years. They also began at the earliest stages with a talented group of professionals, both to deal with the new challenges of the hydrophilic lens, disinfection, and storage, as well as in the delivery of knowledge to professionals. The independence of the ISCLR in relation to manufacturers was not a major issue throughout ISCLR's history, in part because manufacturers participated realizing that such an independent forum benefitted their evaluations of the research status. A review of Appendix 12 shows a variety of Symposium sponsors. Alcon Pharmaceuticals, Allergan Pharmaceuticals, Bausch & Lomb, Cooper Vision(and its predecessors) and Johnson & Johnson(Vistakon) were consistent sponsors to the present from the 1980 or 1982 Symposia. The predominantly gas permeable lens manufacturers were present: Polymer Technology(A division of Bausch & Lomb) in 1980; Paragon Sciences since 2003; and Menicon Co Ltd since 2003.

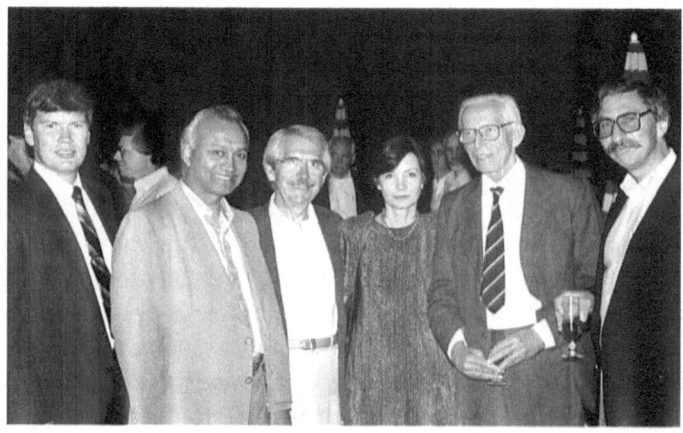

Chemists get together during the Monte Carlo meeting, including invited speaker Danesh Shaw, Miguel Refojo and his wife Svetlana; Otto Wichterle and Buddy Ratner

There have been a large group of company scientists who have substantially contributed throughout ISCLR's history. Many were members: Stuart Eriksen, William Sammons, and Sheldon Wechsler who were Charter members; and later Arthur Back(Cooper Vision), Joseph Barr(B&L), Charles Chandler(B&L), Ian Cox(B&L), Stewart Eriksen(Allergan), Paul Erikson(B&L), Brian Levy(B&L), John McNally (CIBA), George Mertz(J&J), Dorla Mirejovsky(Allergan), Frank Molock (CIBA), Jerry Paugh(Allergan), Cristina Schnider(Menicon), Christopher Snyder(B&L), Ralph Stone(Alcon), and Lynn Winterton (CIBA). Corporate scientists who have contributed to the program throughout this time have also included William Meyers(Paragon), and Kiran Randieri(Alcon).

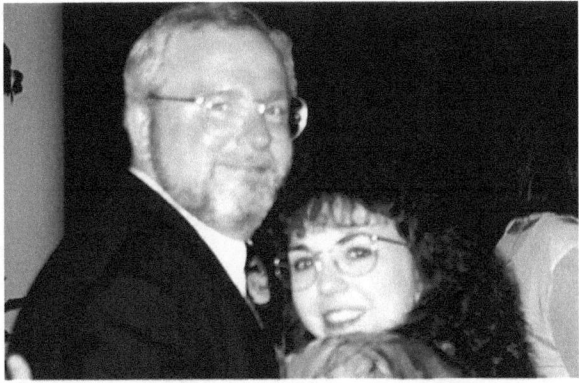

George Mertz represented the highest ideals of a corporate scientist and researcher; with his wife Jill

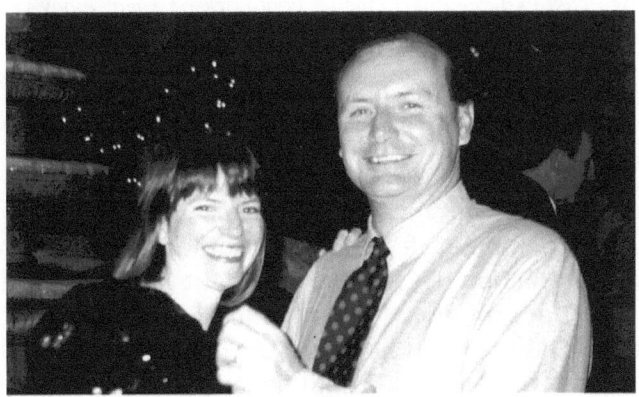

Charlene Gauthier and Timothy Grant's paths cross again as graduate student presenters to respected scientists in the corporate world

A review of the topics during ISCLR's existence show that major research issues appear and reappear. For example, the efficacies of a variety of different solutions were a part of the 1980 London Symposium, and the subject of cleaning efficacy quickly provided the solution manufacturers if not the contact lens manufacturers with possible directions. Also, the bulk and surface properties of contact lens materials are intertwined with the solutions that are intended to keep them efficacious. Possible deficiencies in efficacy of disinfection systems could be similarly followed. Although there may have been hiatuses for various topics, one can only review the Symposium Proceedings of 2005 and 2007 to see that contact lens materials and their solutions interact in different ways with different materials.

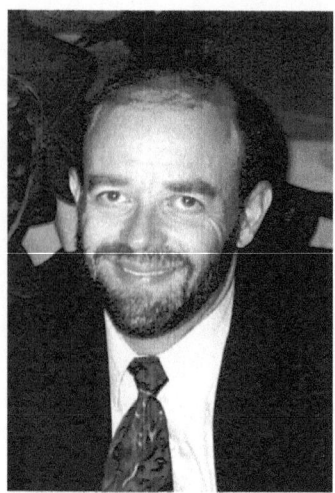

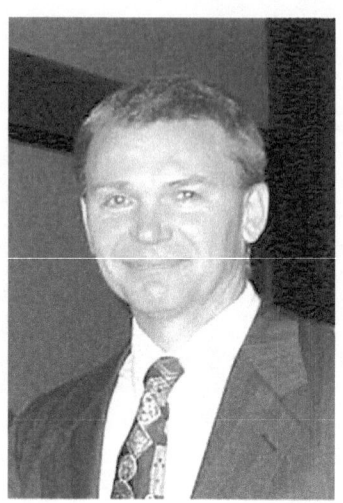

Brian Levy, a researcher in a medical contact lens practice who later went to Bausch & Lomb

Paul Erickson spent many years in industry, took a sabbatical for several years in Sydney, returned to industry, and is once again an Aussie

Despite the predominance of materials science and contact lens solutions at the ISCLR meetings, there is another forum which attempted to expand the interaction. ISCLR Vice President Jean Jacob and Louisiana State University Department of Ophthalmology sponsor the Symposium on the Materials Science and Chemistry of Contact Lenses that are held in New Orleans. The two day symposium began in 1988 in St. Louis where it was first organized by Raymond Myers and the University of Missouri-St. Louis. Since then there have been 14 meetings through which the primary attendees, the chemists and engineers of the corporations meet with academic chemists.

ISCLR and the Materials Science Symposia have created a constructive tension with contact lens manufacturers where some degree of discussion of proprietary information occurs for the benefit of the entire field, perhaps before manufacturers would otherwise release this information. This situation always has existed; but to the degree individual manufacturers have participated in discussing proprietary or embarrassing issues, they have propelled the field in a collaborative way.

The rigid gas permeable field has always provided a critical target for comparison with hydrophilic contact lenses in order to develop a more perfect lens modality. In many ways gas permeable properties were very attractive and they offered the practical contrast which would lead to progress among both modalities. High Dk transmission before soft lens materials, differing extended wear capability, overnight RGP orthokeratology are RGP applications which demonstrate that history is likely to repeat itself at future meetings.

When to go beyond contact lenses; or not?

There has been a periodic controversy whether additional technologies should be included in sessions or in topics that may have an indirect if not remote connection with contact lenses. Examples have included refractive surgery, corneal inlays, and myopia control. A major reason is that a segment of the membership, namely ophthalmology, had associated interests of mutual benefit to the contact lens field. In recent years, optometric and academic members have expanded their research interests into associated areas.

This has manifested itself in panel discussions on refractive surgery in the 90's, but their continuation has not always been close enough to the Society's major focus on contact lens research. Members have argued when this first became an issue in the mid 90's that research specific to refractive surgery should parallel contact lens research topics such as metabolism, wound healing and optics. However, refractive surgery has been included in recent years mostly as a part of the broader topics of priority to contact lens research for that year. To the extent that there is some time set aside for miscellaneous topics, these are also brought up.

Keynote Speakers

Panels that were set up each meeting often included a speaker who set the stage for the subjects that were important at the time. Often, especially in the early meetings, these were members of the society, and they have remained an important resource. But increasingly, the keynote position includes individuals whose research efforts may be relevant, or the next step to advance the contact lens field. Further reasons are to determine how the field might resolve a problem or broaden members' perspectives.

The Board made significant budgetary commitments to bring these outside speakers and encourage them to attend the entire meeting. One of the first was Steven Klyce whose corneal topographical device was new and barely used in contact lens fitting or research. He not only participated with members in developing the topographer to advance contact lens knowledge, but he also contributed from his physiological background and his organizational abilities.

Kenneth Polse summarized ISCLR's ability to bring together a successful group. "I believe that the ISCLR has done a fantastic job in achieving a well-balanced group of investigators and as we develop, we continue to add top scientists to the member rosters. In my opinion this is a very healthy indicator for the society and I think it was at Kauai that this process of adding members with complimentary research began in earnest."

Graduate students and their role in ISCLR

A fortuitous determination as early as the first Symposium was the ISCLR Council was in providing graduate students priority in attendance. In a post evaluation of the 1980 London meeting, Myers said, "Graduate students in contact lens subjects were extremely satisfied with the information and impressed by the gathering of such a body."

At the next Montreal Symposium, four graduate students were invited to attend and the Executive Council decided to reimburse their full and reasonable expenses. Since they were not yet members and were not eligible because of their short careers, this was a departure from the first meetings where the only presentations from non-members aside from keynote speakers were those who had applied for membership. A significant percentage of the budget for up to 15 graduate students was expanded in succeeding years, and most likely contributes to the continued vitality of the Society.

The inclusion of graduate students and keynote speakers had another benefit for future additions to membership. In a closed society, the turnover of officers might be expected to be infrequent. This was a major concern in the early ISCLR, because the Steering Committee did not want to be classified as either an aristocratic or country club type of organization.

"ISCLR has experienced four generations of leadership in its 25 years of existence," Raymond Myers said at the Gala Dinner in the 2005 Coolum Symposium. Myers was referring in part to three age groups which began with one graduate student presenter who went onto the ISCLR Presidency; and a fourth one in Coolum, Australia represented by a graduate student, who was well on her way to distinguishing herself for a future role. The "generations" that Myers defined started with the presidencies of Montague Ruben(1980) and Brien Holden(1982). The second generation manifested itself with Michel Guillon(1997) who attended the first ISCLR's steering committee meeting and presented at the 1980 London Symposium. The third generation began in 1990 when Suzanne Fleiszig from the University of California introduced her novel work on variability in the pseudomonas species. She also held various roles until 2007, when she was elected President.

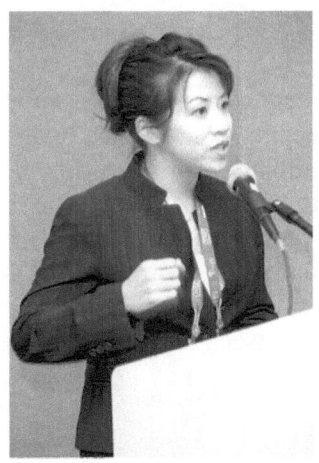

Jennifer Choo moderated a spirited discussion on orthokeratology

To represent an individual at the start of the fourth generation, Myers would not normally encumber a graduate student with such a lofty future. Her deftness in presenting her research combined with mediating a scientific controversy earned her this distinction. Jennifer Choo had as her graduate advisors Brien Holden and Patrick Caroline, and chose to report on a complicated study of overnight gas permeable lens wear in orthokeratology using a cat model. She reported the results in several formats at the 2005 Coolum Caprice meeting which included a delivered presentation. After her presentation, Choo found herself leading a discussion that had much broader significance than her research. A scientific paradox surfaced following the recent approval of the FDA of an overnight wear lens in contrast to a recent publication by Helen Swarbrick presenting a meta-analysis of serious complications of overnight wear in orthokeratology in Asia. Choo deftly moderated this controversy that was based upon Swarbrick's findings and the formidable international authorities in epidemiology of Oliver Schein, Fiona Stapleton, Noel Dilly, and Helen Swarbrick.

The reactions of the graduate students to presenting at the ISCLR have run a spectrum of expectations. Choo who was early in her graduate studies commented that she gained confidence in her presentation by the grasp of her research area. Her familiarity with those in other fields had just begun which lessened any apprehension. Suzanne Fleiszig's memory in her presentation, and also a graduate student who had completed her requirements, was of Dwight Cavanagh, the moderator of the session, and the awe in presenting to the assembly of individuals she knew through their publications. She was part of a group of graduate students at the 1990 Monte Carlo symposium consisting of Helen Swarbrick and Fiona Stapleton where she recalls having met the two for the first time despite all being from Australia. Fleiszig studied with Nathan

Efron and Noel Brennan in Melbourne and finished her PhD also spending 6 months with Gerald Pier.

Richard Hill has been responsible for the expansion and the success of this program throughout the years. This included heading a subcommittee of the Executive Council who read and prioritized the abstracts and selected many of the participants. A poster session was developed, and in itself has become an important addition to the Symposia. Not only have the students had the opportunity to discuss their findings with members during the session breaks, but the posters stimulate another route for member interactions throughout the Symposia. Hill also instituted a session on the last day for questions and further discussion.

Transcript Publication

The Proceedings of the Symposia probably have made the greatest transformation through ISCLR history than any other aspect. First, the time in preparing them was enormous compared to its potential use, and the Council revisited their need very frequently. Second, the format for these has changed from doing a transcript of the audiotape to today's modern version of a digital disk combining the Power Point slides with written summaries. Third, the transcripts have forced meeting organizers to summarize the sessions, and the information became a better summary for the members and the sponsoring corporations.

The editors during the early meetings through 1986 were Kenneth Polse with the assistance of Michel Guillon. Thereafter, the Sydney group through Deborah Sweeney carried out the publication. The transcripts continued until Hayman Islands(1993) when a mixture of presentation summaries and transcripts. As early as Phuket(1999) the proceedings consisted of summaries and Power Point slides.

There has always been feedback from members that the transcripts are useful. They are intentionally for members use, and are not citable. Also, at least the Executive Council believed they were obliged to provide the sponsored manufacturers the CD or publication because of the staff at their offices would want to review these. Technology has facilitated the presentation of something that is more manageable today; they are also a part of the summaries of the sessions, and most presenters and moderators are attuned to ISCLR's publication and session form.

Suzanne Fleiszig recalls the influence that the Proceedings had on her, when she first went as a graduate student to the 1990 meeting. She was provided an earlier transcript to read before she went. She became entranced by it, not only for the information, but in the conversations among the participants. The process of idea development in these conversations was a major part of her analysis and interest. In later years when she was called upon to moderate the sessions and later prepare the proceedings, she remembers the impact the transcripts had on her, and has personally added transcripts from her moderated sessions.

Persistence of Topics and Debate through Various Symposia

It is beyond the scope of this book to follow the history of the many topics that have surfaced and resurfaced during the 30 year history of ISCLR. The availability online to ISCLR members of the Programs and Proceedings of fourteen Symposia make it comparatively easy to follow topics and either through the Programs, the Proceedings, or the speaker presentations for the different panels.

However, one of the early issues, oxygen transmissibility through contact lenses, illustrates the mechanisms through which the ISCLR debated and carried through with a difficult problem. On a chronological basis, Nathan Efron describes what he terms "the Dk Wars." As Nathan describes, the ISCLR instituted a new vehicle, an interest group, who met specifically to standardize a method for researchers to report Dk through different measurement methods.

The starting point for the Dk War was in the mid-1980s with a small article in the UK weekly magazine Ophthalmic Optician, claiming that the Dk value of a new rigid gas permeable fluoro-silicone-acrylate lens, manufactured by 3M, was 170. The problem was that the ocular response to this lens—in particular the amount of closed-eye corneal edema induced by this lens—was not commensurate Fatt's claimed Dk value. This created particular difficulties because Irv was the doyen of Dk measurement and few felt motivated to challenge him on this.

However, at that time, Noel Brennan and I had commenced measuring Dk using Fatt's polarographic techniques and found lower values for the 3M lens, although our values were somewhat unreliable. Further research suggested that Irv Fatt's initial inflated value could be attributed to what became known as edge effects and boundary effects. Other labs around the world started wading into the argument, and it was Brien Holden who, at the 5th ISCLR meeting in 1988 in Hawaii, suggested that multiple but identical sets of 'standard' lenses be developed and sent to all interested labs for measurement. This was done, with the great Irv Fatt's 'blessing', and two years later an important paper was published, leading to an international consensus. This paper is:

Holden BA, Newton-Howes J, Winterton L, Fatt I, Hamano H, LaHood D, Brennan NA, Efron N. The Dk project: An interlaboratory comparison of Dk/L measurements. Optom Vis Sci: 1990; 67(6): 476-481.

The publication of this work led to a refinement of the International Standard for Dk measurement, which specifically laid out approaches for edge and boundary corrections. Since that time, there has been good agreement between Dk values reported by industry and reported independent laboratories. This is especially evident today in the context of silicone hydrogel lenses, whereby all reported values for these products over the past decade since their introduction have been in general agreement.

Efron believes that this example illustrates the significant role that the ISCLR plays in bringing about a consensus on a difficult issue. There are other examples some that are discussed next by Miguel Refojo where the ISCLR becomes a timely forum for resolving difficult issues and reaching a consensus. "Even if the ISCLR through its limited mission of holding periodic meeting does not have the conduit to resolve difficult issues, it is a platform for open debate and discussion that has pointed the way forward," says Efron.

Miguel Refojo commented on the Dk war from the standpoint of the polymer chemist controversy. He also demonstrates just within the chemistry field the wide variety of topics that have been included throughout the many Symposia. He also distinguishes how similar issues starting in 1980 are likely to be discussed at the 2009 Crete Symposium.

A fundamental difference between the original rigid PMMA contact lenses and the new soft HEMA hydrogel lenses was the water content of the hydrogel. This contributed not only to the comfort of the lens, but also to their oxygen permeability, a very important property for the corneal health. However, it was soon realized that the oxygen transmissibility of the HEMA hydrogel lenses was insufficient to satisfy cornea requirements. Therefore, new hydrogels lenses of higher hydration than PHEMA, made of copolymers of hydrophilic monomers with or without HEMA that increased their oxygen permeability.

Concurrently, a persistent topic of discussion at the Society meetings have been the methods of measurement of oxygen permeability of contact lenses materials, and ultimately the oxygen transmissibility of specific lenses in relation to the oxygen demand of the cornea, with and without lenses, and with open or closed eyes. The method and results of the determination of oxygen demand of the cornea has been also an important topic of discussion.

With the early realization of the importance of the oxygen permeability for contact lens material, the search among available polymers with known oxygen permeability and good optical properties was easily focused in silicone rubber. Various laboratories, at least in the USA, Japan and France, produced silicone elastomeric contact lenses. As far as oxygen transmissibility is concerned they were ideal, and the problem of hydrophobicity was also taken care by surface modification, by plasma polymerization or by radiation grafting for example. Nevertheless, the ultimate failure of the silicone elastomeric lenses was due to their tendency to adhere to the cornea, and its consequences. The mechanism of adhesion of these lenses to the cornea was studied and discussed often. The predominant opinion of the cause of adhesion of silicone elastomeric lenses to the cornea was the so-called suction-cup effect, despite the fact that even when flatter lenses, fitted with mobility on the cornea, also tended to adhere. Another possible factor of adhesion was the already known high water perevaporation through silicone rubber membranes that, in the case of the contact lenses, resulted in the loss of the water.

Other possible causes of these problems of contact lens adhesion could have related to the tacky nature of the surface of silicone rubber. Also, a commercial failure was that a semisoft contact lens made essentially of a copolymer containing polyperfluoropolyether moieties, had good oxygen permeability and wettability, but finally could not compete with the standard hydrogel contact lenses.

Parallel to the development of new hydrogel soft contact lenses was that of rigid gas permeable lenses, heir to the PMMA lenses. Several lenses were made of commercial polymers with some degree of oxygen permeability, but not sufficient for successful contact lenses. However, the introduction of a truly oxygen permeable rigid contact lens (RGP) made of a copolymer of MMA with a siloxane-methacrylate (TRIS) as principal ingredients, was invented by chemist Norman Gaylord, in collaboration of the optometrist Leonard Seidner. Then, several new RGP contact lenses followed based on the same chemistry, with more or less modification on the formulation of the copolymer, but always with TRIS or a TRIS like oxygen permeable moieties.

Now we are in the era of the siloxane-hydrogel contact lenses, consisting of hybrid copolymers with hydrophilic moieties from hydrogel materials, and hydrophobic organosilicon moieties from silicone elastomeric lenses and/or the TRIS siloxane monomers similar to RGP lens materials. These lenses are usually named silicone-hydrogels which is only correct if they contain silicone moieties, that it is a polysiloxane {-Si-O-Si-O-Si-O-} backbone.

However, if the contact lens material contains as it principal oxygen permeable moiety a TRIS like monomer with carbon to carbon backbone {C-C-C-} and siloxane {-Si-O} radicals in side branches, it is then incorrect to name them silicone-hydrogel. On the other hand, in both cases, with silicone or TRIS-like moieties, the denomination siloxane-hydrogel will be the correct one. Is this semantics? No, not for chemists. A good argument for an ISCLR meeting.

The siloxane-hydrogel lenses are a new class of contact lenses materials, with excellent oxygen permeability and good wear comfort. However, as with any new kind of contact lenses, the early claims are usually very positive, but with the passage of time and the amount of lenses by a variety of persons and different ambient conditions increase, problems might occur. Under other recurrent topics of discussion not related to corneal hypoxia, are other complications of contact lens wear, possibly produced by toxic, immunological or mechanical causes. Tear film and surface wettability of contact lenses, water evaporation from the eye with and without contact lenses, and tear protein and lipids deposits on the lenses and their effect on bacteria adhesion and biofilm formation on the lenses and its relation to bacterial keratitis are often discussed at the ISCLR meetings.

Under other recurrent topics of discussion not related to corneal hypoxia, are other complications of contact lens wear, possibly produced by toxic, immunological or mechanical causes. Tear film and surface wettability of contact lenses, water evaporation from the eye with and without contact lenses, and tear protein and lipids deposits on the lenses and their effect on bacteria adhesion and biofilm formation on the lenses and its relation to bacterial keratitis are often discussed at the ISCLR meetings.

Chapter 5

Symposia

2nd Symposium—Montreal, Canada— September 1-3, 1982

The 1982 Montreal Symposium although it was the second symposium actually became the model for future meetings. Brien Holden was chair and Michel Guillon was the conference secretary. The topics are the starting points followed by a series of questions or issues that are to be addressed. Members receive the topics about 9 months before the next symposium and are asked to contribute abstracts considering the meeting focuses. Initially, it was expected at the early meetings that most all would provide an abstract until the focus was changed to the major topics. Members were not necessarily expected to make a presentation in later meetings.

Montreal was selected as the meeting location to facilitate the attendance for Americans, because the ophthalmologist contingency asked that the first meetings avoid locating in the United States. ISCLR's beginning in America was auspicious because there was a significant degree of interest and knowledge about the proposed International Contact Lens Association and the eventual International Society for Contact Lens Research. Whereas a research society resolved much of the conflict with European ophthalmology, it actually created problems in America in part because of the differing individuals who would be members of a research society. Refojo recently stated the obvious: "the interdisciplinary composition of the ISCLR is fundamental." However, just before the Symposium in Montreal small crises took place when ophthalmology cadres pressured their colleagues not to participate at professional meetings with optometrists. Perry Binder recalls, "As a Board member of CLAO, I was told it would have been inappropriate to attend a meeting of Optometrists. However, most ophthalmologists that were members decided not to obey and continued as active members of the Society." This influenced attendance in Montreal, and Michael Lemp was the only one who came. His presence was in fact representative of the others(9 altogether) who would be at subsequent meetings. Montreal represented the most difficult multiprofessional situation and was a turning point because the results showed the seriousness of a scientific meeting for the membership without public fanfare.

The issues of the time included the first day with two sessions devoted to the tears from its structure and function to tear interaction with the lens. Frank Holly was one of the people of the time who contributed extensively to the meeting. The third session was on Materials development with the two major issues being gas permeable rigid lenses and high water content and their properties. Among those contributing were Miguel Refojo as the Keynote Speaker of the session with Buddy Ratner and his bioengineering focus. The remaining subjects for the last three sessions were the contact lens effects on the eye, extended wear contact lenses, and lens design and behavior.

Epiphanies do not ordinarily occur in science, but Michel Guillon recalls Ratner's presentation on the connections between surface protein deposition and lens materials which later defined the four group FDA Classification for Hydrogels.

ISCLR Charter membership was determined by applicants applying for membership through 1982. Before this, membership was sparse and not yet representative. Therefore, the Council chose to define the Charter membership by the applications which began in 1980 and extended to before the meeting in 1982. This numbered 87 Charter Members listed in Appendix 3.

The Montreal site was chosen for its pleasant ambiance at this time of year. Myers and Guillon worked together toward making arrangements as well as carrying out the program set by the Chairperson Brien Holden and Executive Committee. The position of Secretary-Treasurer held by Myers was in fact subdivided into the Vice President-Finance which Myers continued to hold for 15 years, and Guillon became the secretary.

For the Montreal meeting Myers was designated as the officer to make hotel arrangements including the Gala Dinner and its menu. The dinner was thought to blend the ambiance of the French Canadian cuisine with getting out of the hotel for its social and relaxing benefits. Myers knew this would be a precarious position because Guillon's French birth upbringing had been barely influenced by a decade of living in the UK. Perhaps the best way to characterize Myers and Guillon's close working relationship until then and for the next 15 years was to look at the national rivalry between the French and the Americans during that time period.

A couple of days before everyone arrived, Myers went to the restaurant to choose the menu. Through considerable discussion with the owner and some taste testing, he made a selection of foods that were Québécois and also represented acceptable cuisine for an international attendance. Two selections apparently without a basis in French cuisine were Myers' choice of the soup and the dessert. The soup translated to English was "cold watermelon soup" and the dessert was "fresh strawberries with cream AND cracked black pepper." The dinner attendees appeared to be pleasantly surprised and satisfied with the selections. Guillon with Myers' help never did forget the evident discordance with French food.

3rd Symposium—Cambridge, England— September 23-25, 1984

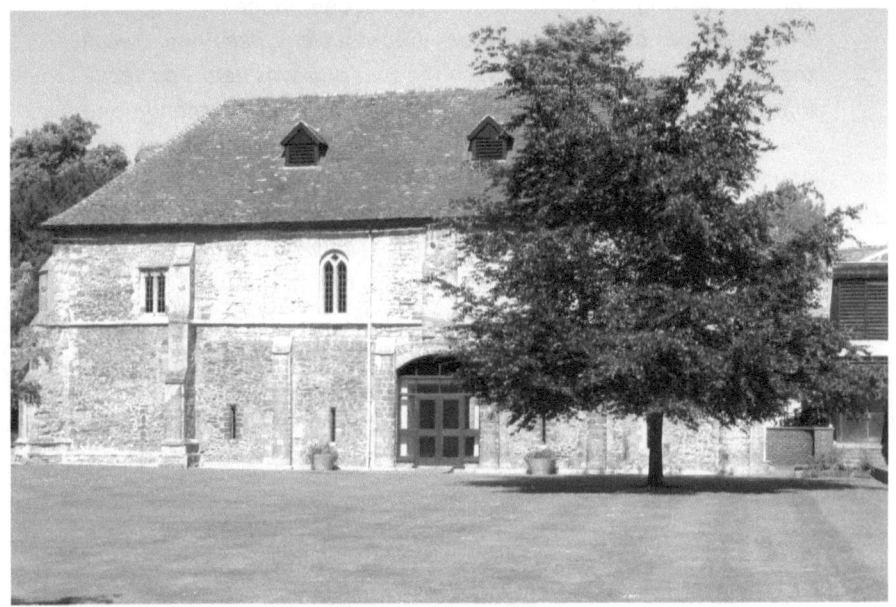

The School of Pathagoros was the site of the 1984 Symposium and a part of St. John's College of Cambridge University

Cambridge University was chosen as the third symposium site for this fledging society. Among various sites at the university was the Pythagorean Hall at St. John's College which resembled internally a small church with an open hall. Miguel Refojo was ISCLR President and Meeting Co-Chairmen were Kenneth Polse and Brien Holden. Holden introduced St. John's College as follows:

We are pleased to meet here in St. John's Cambridge in the Pythagorean Hall, which was rebuilt recently from ruins that were here since 1200. I understand that this was the domicile of the people who lived here at the time, and downstairs was where they kept the pigs and the sheep. So if you need a meeting place for Australians or others, it is downstairs.

As distinguished as the site was, the cool temperature in Cambridge was not conducive to the meeting except to keep the audience awake. In addition, the availability of rooms was such that the Council arranged Graduate housing, which although modern and acceptable by many standards did not reach the conveniences that some of the attendees were used to. Upon spending one night in the rooms, Irvin Borish, Maurice Poster and their wives started the exodus to downtown hotels which with short notice, were sparse. Some endured including new attendee Stephen Klyce.

> *The first meeting I attended was the third in Cambridge meeting as an invited speaker by one of my heroes in contact lens, Ken Polse. I recall the stone meeting room in which the meeting was held—perfectly informal for the society style that encouraged easy exchange and discussion. I also recall the student housing. My room was so cold I purchased sweaters in which I slept. The day before I left, I think someone on the staff finally realized a poor spoiled white lad was staying there and cracked the hidden heat valve just a bit so that my bath towel was slightly less than soggy in the morning.*

Perry Binder recalled, "I too was cold the entire time I tried to sleep in the dorm. Only one small postage stamp towel was available and I had to dry it on the small wall radiator between uses. It had to last four days! Sleeping was also difficult because the walls and ceilings were paper thin; one could hear EVERY thing in adjacent rooms."

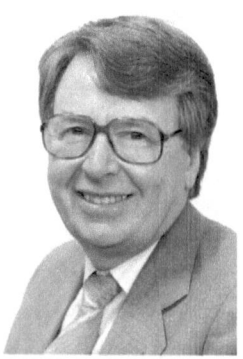

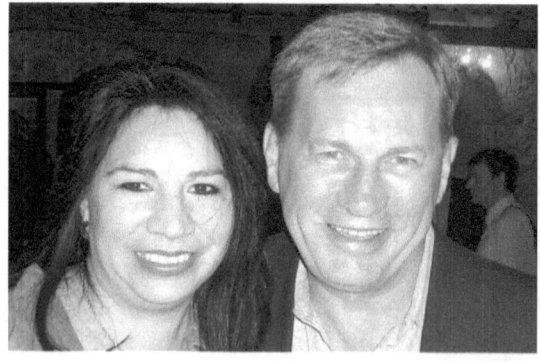

Brian Tighe became increasingly involved in contact lens polymers and most recently is an ISCLR Vice President

Since 1984, Jan Bergmanson has consistently reported on the microstructures of contact lens materials and wearing effects. His wife Peggy has often accompanied him

The facilities actually were conducive for the creation of many of the methods that are used today to gain maximal interaction in discussion. Holden declared in his introductory remarks. "The philosophy that originated the International Society for Contact Lens Research and was confirmed again by the Council meeting yesterday is that this Society is a closed society for elected members as a sort of international think tank discussion." The open environment of St. John's College allowed Holden and Guillon to arrange and rearrange seating during the breaks to improve interaction, in addition to persuading moderators to minimize presentations with more interaction. Thirty years later, Kenneth Polse notes as follows:

"A significant memory was the Cambridge meeting. It was a great meeting. All the necessary components were present; the leading scientists in contact lens/corneal physiology, outstanding graduate students who aspired to a career in contact lens research, collegiality, cutting edge discussions among the group and a venue that was inspiring and appropriate for this meeting. One could not possibly have attended the Cambridge ISLCR meeting and leave without the feeling that the Society was a fantastic conduit for discussion and encouragement of contact lens research."

Among the important topics of the meeting was the first session led by Montague Ruben on optical performance and image quality. A distinguished group of individuals led by Melvin Freeman as keynote speaker, and Arthur Bennett, Guenter Forst, William Sammons, Robert Mandell, and Michel Millodot created a stimulating session. On the next day, the entire day was devoted to the topic, "Effects of Daily and Extended Wear Contact Lenses on the Cornea" at a time when extended wear was being evaluated compared to daily wear as an alternative form of wear.

The ISCLR Council gradually developed a plan to alternate meetings between Europe, North America, and Australia and the Far East. ISCLR was an international organization, with substantial contributors in each of these regions, so that different areas were necessary to retain and to expand its international character. Another characteristic was to hold the meeting in a warm climate where there was at least some possibility to recover from the rigors of the meeting which was to expand to a 3 ½ day meeting at the next 1986 meeting in S'Agaro. There continued to be some falloff of attendance in some of the sessions that were not necessarily related to individuals' direct research pursuits, but this became less of an issue with the better use of interactive discussions first with the panels, and then with more enthusiastic audience inclusion.

An ISCLR Executive Council meeting was held during the American Academy of Optometry(AAO) in St. Louis in December, 1984. The was an auspicious meeting because this began the string of 26 annual Australian Parties at the AAO first sponsored by the Corneal & Contact Lens Unit of the University of New South Wales. Myers whose practice was in St. Louis made the local arrangements including scouring the home city of Budweiser Beer for every can of Fosters Ale. True to life, this did not dissuade Brien Holden who because of the resounding success of the first party, wanted to hold a second Australian party the next night! Myers again scoured the city, knowing that the Budweiser Beer City would be able to handle Holden's insatiable wishes.

The ISCLR Executive Council met at a dinner meeting at Myers' house. The meeting was otherwise conventional except Myers had other activity at his house. Myers' wife Paulette was building a metalsmithing program at the nearby university. Her efforts were interrupted because the roof of her freestanding building separated. In order to continue the program and after two unsuccessful locations on campus, she volunteered the garage of their home which began the official studio of the university for her 15+ students. The ISCLR Council met on a night during the week of final examinations for the students, so the meeting and dinner proceeded with frequent hammering in the basement and the adjoining garage. Rather than being a diversion, the two groups finally came together after the meeting and dinner, and the students already had attracted an international audience.

4ᵗʰ Symposium—S 'Agaro, Spain—September 15-18, 1986

S'Agaro, Spain was a tropical venue recommended by Antonio Henriquez whose vacation home was nearby, and Monty Ruben who was building a retirement home there. The group met at a small but lavish hotel, Hotel La Gavina that accommodated most of the society. The environment could be described as a verdant area in a valley facing the Mediterranean Sea where the prevailing winds would normally produce rain once a day, between midnight until dawn. This was ISCLR's first meeting in a tropical environment where each day the meeting would extend from 9:00 AM-7:30PM, but included a long period—2-2 ½ hours in the middle of the day—with relatively free time for participants to rest and relax in the outdoors. This schedule was in sharp contrast to the Montreal and Cambridge schedule where the consensus was that continuously meeting without a break was particularly grueling.

Miguel Refojo was President and Kenneth Polse was the Program Chair. The first two sessions in Montreal were a "Free Papers" section headed by Brien Holden and an Anatomy and Physiology session with moderator Stephen Klyce. Much of the day was in discussion of various corneal structures including the endothelial role in corneal function. One half day was spent on refractive surgery with Perry Binder heading the session where Klyce discussed corneal topography, and Roger Buckley described "excimer laser keratoplasty." Other half day sessions were devoted to Ocular & Contact Lens Surfaces with Miguel Refojo as moderator; Lens Materials and Properties with Donald Korb; Contact Lens Visual Performance with Michel Guillon; and Ocular Pharmacology,

Toxicology, and Immunology with Montague Ruben. A highlight was a spirited discussion referenced earlier by Miguel Refojo and Nathan Efron on the disparity in measurement methods of oxygen. Other interesting presentations included a' video presentation by Marshall Doane, whose cinematography with high speed photography demonstrated novel tear film mechanisms. Also, Drahoslov Lim, cohort to Otto Wichterle in the first hydrophilic patent, and currently living in the US was at the meeting.

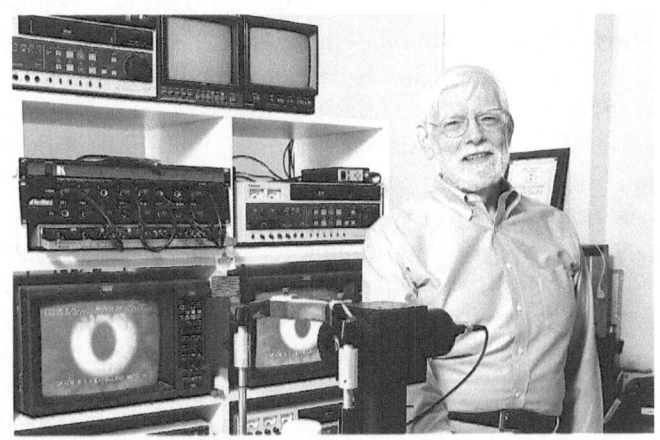

Marshal Doane produced some of the earliest and most sophisticated videos of high speed tear film and lens movement

Hans Bleshoy, Joseph Bonanno, Arthur Ho and Steve Kwok received funding equivalent to members traveling from the same region of the world. The Council also adopted a policy that would remain thereafter. Members who have not attended the past two meetings would be subject to forfeiture of membership. The obvious purpose was to keep the most active researchers within the limited membership society and to recognize that the Symposium was the predominant benefit and responsibility for membership.

An important juncture occurred at the Executive Council meeting when the location of the next meeting was discussed and the decision was to go to Hawaii. ISCLR had a concentration of meetings in Europe because of the inability to meet in the US. Considering the international representation of ISCLR members, there was a compelling need to hold future meeting in other regions. Australian members were anxious to hold a future meeting, but the costs seemed prohibitive. Hawaii became an option and the major advantage was inexpensive airfares compared with locations in the Asian Pacific. As the Executive Council came close to recommending Hawaii, Ray Myers and Montague Ruben exchanged incredulous glances. Myers recalled to the Board the earlier history of scheduling a meeting in the US. Directing his remarks to the two American ophthalmologists Michael Lemp and Perry Binder, he asked "has ISCLR now passed the interprofessional difficulties of the earlier years?" and they agreed was that we had.

Deborah Sweeney has concluded what members learned until now and has been the strength of ISCLR through the present. "It has always been said that better friendships and less politics exist in research."

"1986 was an interesting year for me," recalls Perry Binder. "As chairman of the Cornea Section of ARVO, I instituted the first Contact Lens topical session. As the President of the Contact Lens Association of Ophthalmologists, I invited Brien Holden to debate me on the advantages and disadvantages of Extended Wear Contact Lenses. Needless to say, I took a lot of "heat" from the establishment for inviting an Optometrist as a guest lecturer, but the session was very well attended in the January, 1986, meeting in Las Vegas."

The S'Agaro meeting was memorable to Treasurer Ray Myers for learning the vagaries of Spanish financial transactions. Unlike other countries, it was not easy or safe to transfer payments for local expenses for which ISCLR was responsible. Another complication was that the American dollar was slipping relative to European currencies because Saadam Hussein was saber rattling days before he would enter Kuwait. Henriquez suggested that Myers make an electronic wire transfer of US$10,000 to Henriquez' account and his bank branch in Barcelona. When Myers arrived in Barcelona, Henriquez and Myers went to the bank and found there was no transfer nor could they locate it from documents brought by Myers. By the next morning, the authorization had not surfaced, so Henriquez lent the ISCLR $10,000, which he delivered in a bundle of 2,000,000 pesetas! By the end of the day, he contacted Myers to say the authorization had finally appeared and he had another 2,000,000 pesetas. The assumptions was that it would be safe because Myers would deposit it in the hotel safety deposit box and Henriquez would take him the next day to S'Agaro. However, when Myers asked the hotel agent for a safety deposit box, he kept the packages because the night receptionist held the one and only key of the safety box. That night, Myers spent a restless night in his room with 4,000,000 Pts under his pillow! The challenge did not end until Myers figured out how to spend the excess pesetas in S'Agaro.

The ambiance of this location was unique perhaps because it was the first tropical choice and with Henriquez' role in the location, hotel, and the dinner functions. A Spanish night was held at Blandas, Costa Brava, a ½ hour private bus ride on a circuitous, and beautiful hilly road overlooking the sea. Stephen Klyce, although he was at Cambridge found this meeting particularly memorable. "That was where I really met Ray

Myers. Somehow I ended up sharing a rather large bottle of scotch with him one night on the room patio. While solving the ills of the world, we became fast friends."

Such personal experiences were repeated many times in quickly bringing Steve and others' expertise into to the challenges of the contact lens field.

5th Symposium—Kauai, USA—1988—August 31-September 3, 1988

The Kauai meeting was a memorable meeting in terms in the ambiance of the location and in its contribution to the overall development of the society. Kenneth Polse, ISCLR President that year said, "I have good memories of the meeting in Kauai. It was during that period that soft lens science started to come together and it was possible to more easily understand and appreciate the excitement of contact lens science. I remember that the Kauai represented an expansion of our membership in terms of expertise and diversity. The Board wanted to include not only scientists whose background was in optometry of ophthalmology, but also those scientists who had training outside of vision science and would be able to add and complement to the overall quality of contact lens science."

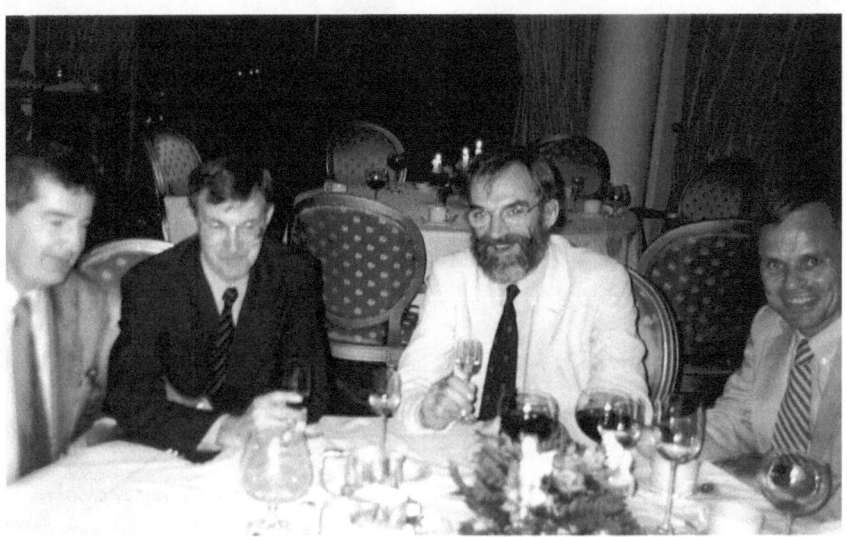

Daniel O' Leary, Leo Carney, Graeme Wilson, and graduate student John Laurent

Chairperson for this meeting was Richard Hill whose program emphasized the ocular surface and its physiology, anatomy, and its effects upon optical performance. Assessment of materials properties and performance were also included along with the effects of care systems on ocular performance. At the S'Agaro meeting, a study committee was developed to try and resolve the variability in generally accepted oxygen measurement techniques and the report was given by Nathan Efron, Irvin Fatt, and others. The committee also consisting of manufacturers' representation with Lynn Winterton of CIBA Vision developed a series of standard contact lenses that would allow oxygen measurements from different labs. Other highlights of the meeting included Mathea Allensmith's explanation of the lid reactions to lens deposits which were continuing as a problem of the time. Another highlight was the discussion of current frontiers of instrumentation led by Kenneth Polse and Stephen Klyce which included Buddy Ratner's ESCA electron spectroscopy application to soft contact lens surfaces. Barry Masters discussed the confocal microscope which would receive even more interest with Masters and Dwight Cavanagh at the next symposium.

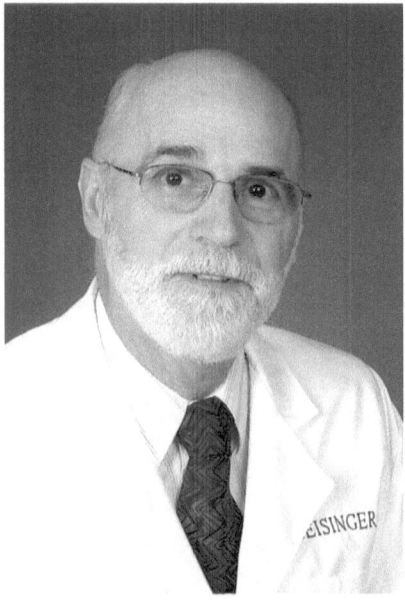

A member since 1988, Donald Egan conducts his research in a medical department setting

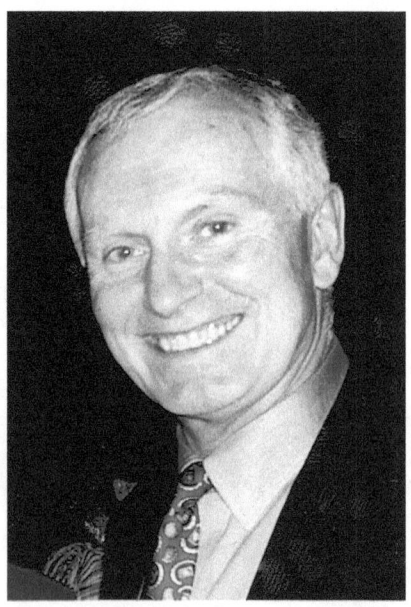

Charter member Charles McMonnies has participated at each ISCLR meeting.

Kauai was an attractive site for the meeting being held at the Waiohai Hotel at Poipu Beach. The small island extended from very dry to extreme rainfall(several hundred inches per year) in different regions of the island. This was a four day meeting without a long break so during the meeting, much of the time was spent around the hotel during the long lunch time breaks. However, the Gala Dinner was held in the outdoor gardens and swimming pool area where Dr. Richard Hill was installed as president. After the formalities, new attendee and member Jerry Paugh recalls the after dinner party and his initiation to the informality and collegiality of the Society. Accompanied by his significant other and future wife Loma, he recalls that the after party continued near the swimming pool where Brien Holden decided to bring some life into the austere group remaining, consisting of Nathan Efron in a new white suit, Raymond Myers, Michel Guillon, and a few others. Before he left, all of them ended up in the swimming pool, with help from Holden. Paugh's newness and perhaps his spouse kept him from joining the hydrated group. Efron remembers, "Jerry and Noel laughed at me later as I carefully ironed my US$20 bills in my hotel room because all my money was soaked!"

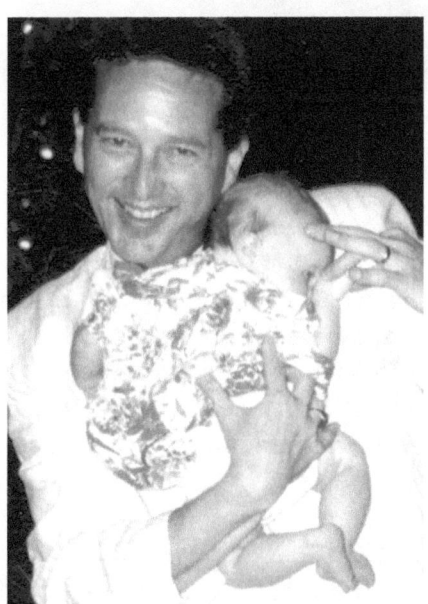

Nathan Efron, in his white suit which lasted only through the Kauai symposium, prepares a next generation candidate for ISCLR membership

6th Symposium—Monte Carlo, Monaco: August 31-September 3, 1990

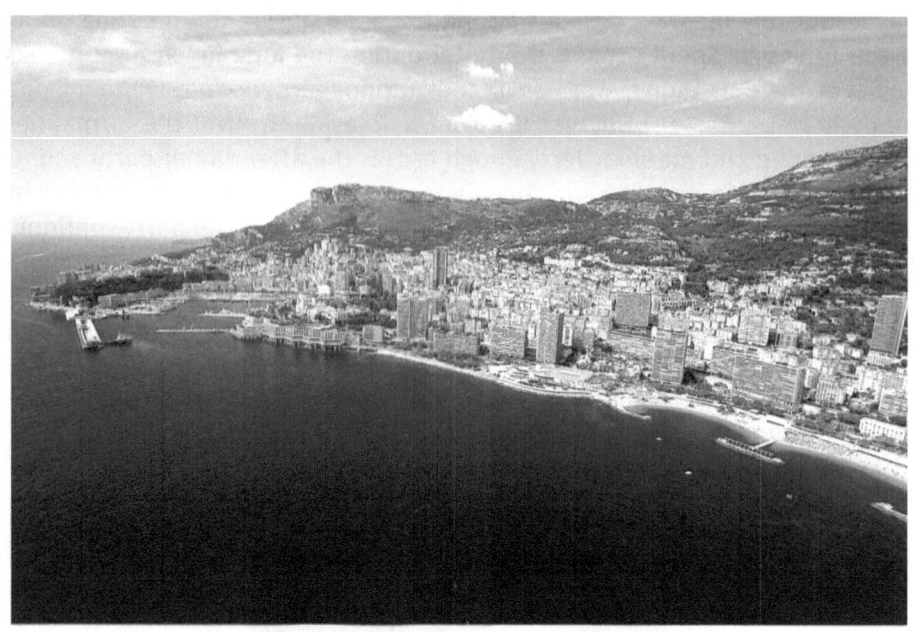

The Monte Carlo Symposium(1980)

The 1990 Monaco Symposium became the first concerted implementation of bringing outside researchers at a time when the contact lens field was in a state of transition, between new materials and with greater challenges in newer areas. Consequently, there were five keynote speakers, two were new to the ISCLR. They were Danesh Shah and Richard Lembach. The existing members were Brian Tighe, Donald Korb, and Dwight Cavanagh with two keynote presentations because of standing in for another keynote speaker could not attend. Also, two non-members, Jay Krachmer and Noel Dilly, were also there as moderators and contributors.

Richard Hill was the ISCLR President and Michael Lemp was the Program Chair. The subjects covered a variety of problems in both hydrogels and rigid lenses. Buddy Ratner, Michel Guillon, and Cristina Schnider explored bulk vs. surface properties. Possible considerations of changing the surface properties were being proposed as a possible solution to some of these problems.

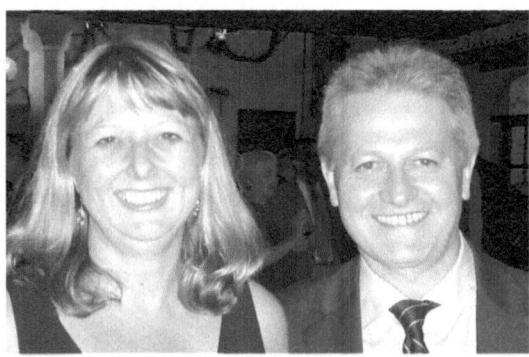

Deborah Sweeney takes Michel Guillon's position after
8 years as ISCLR Secretary

Dwight Cavanagh attending his first meeting provided a considerable contribution in Monte Carlo with two keynote presentations, one on the first confocal microscope and the second, contact lens related ocular immunology. The confocal presentation was a lengthy result of an international collaboration, and the use of this new paradigm for high magnification of the living cornea was becoming a reality. In the same session graduate student Suzanne Fleiszig and Brian Levy identified the challenging the microbiological problems that were occurring in the contact lens field.

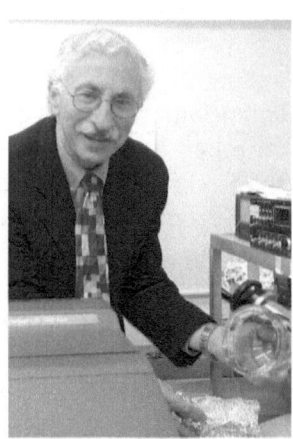

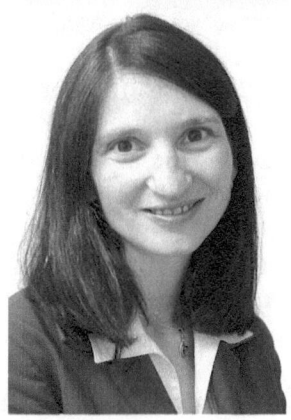

Buddy Ratner's pursuits within contact lens science were always substantial and he was a continual contributor despite many other research and administrative responsibilities

Fiona Staplelton as a graduate student presenter in 1990 began her substantial contributions to this and succeeding meetings

William Meyers, representing a manufacturer scientist, reminded delegates with constructive criticism of the effects in certain actions on manufacturers.

> *Speaking as a lens manufacturer, it is sometimes frustrating for manufacturers like me at meetings like this, because I don't think you realize the importance of the guidance that comes out of this meeting. Let me give two examples: It is noteworthy how little mention has been made during this meeting of the 3M lens—the Advent lens. This was a major topic of discussion at the previous meeting. Things have obviously changed; the lens has not done well. Yet I think the people who brought this lens to market had good reason to think that it was strongly endorsed, at least clinically (certainly not officially), by many of you.*
>
> *Another example was the discussion of disposable lenses that has gone on at this meeting suggests that disposable daily wear may be the mode of choice for many of the practitioners here. I make no judgment about these lenses or the implied endorsement other than to say: let's not kid ourselves. Disposables are being sold for convenience and extended wear, and all the talk we do in this meeting is not likely to change.*
>
> *I simply state this so you are aware that what you say about these lens modalities makes a lot of difference to the manufacturers. My challenge is simply that everyone makes sure their words are properly understood.*

Otto Wichterle attended the Monte Carlo meeting with two of his graduate students. Since the London Symposium, Wichterle had a very difficult time to travel, as he did at other times of his life. In the Soviet Union's occupation of Czechoslovakia, scientific organizations attempted to marginalize his preeminent position. Czech leaders in science at this time obtained their position through their Communist connections. Wichterle's scientific success and his role in humanitarian causes, earning him the title of "Czechoslovakian Sakharov," made him impatient with Soviet dogma and inefficiencies.

Nevertheless, Wichterle received permission from the Communist government to travel to Monte Carlo at the Board's invitation and was to be provided a stipend for him and his students. However, before the ISCLR meeting, the Soviets left Czechoslovakia as they had or would in other countries. As ISCLR Vice President-Finance, Myers was Wichterle's intermediary. He was prepared to transfer the funds to Dr. Wichterle, and at the time communication was best handled over the telephone. Wichterle had what few citizens were allowed which were two bank accounts at the same bank: one for his transactions in Czechoslovakian currency and the other for US dollar transactions. Wichterle explained how the official exchange rate with the US dollar was so low as to make the converted funds nearly worthless. He then provided the bank number of his US dollar account to transfer money by wire.

In Monte Carlo, he arrived and soon Myers confirmed if he had received the transfer. He said that he had not, so Myers produced the wire transfer papers. He compared the papers with his information, and suddenly Wichterle became pale! He had noted that the wire transfer went to his Czech currency account which he had given Myers over the telephone erroneously. He was concerned that the money given the Communist regulations was lost, but he could not do anything until he returned. The Board heard this story and without any hesitation agreed to reimburse him again if he did not receive the full stipend. After the meeting Wichterle did not call so he called him. Wichterle had not called because despite the mistake, he received the full stipend. Because the communists were NO longer in control, civility had begun to return when a helpful bank officer intercepted the transfer and placed it in his US currency account.

7th Symposium—Hayman Island, Australia: September 6-10, 1993

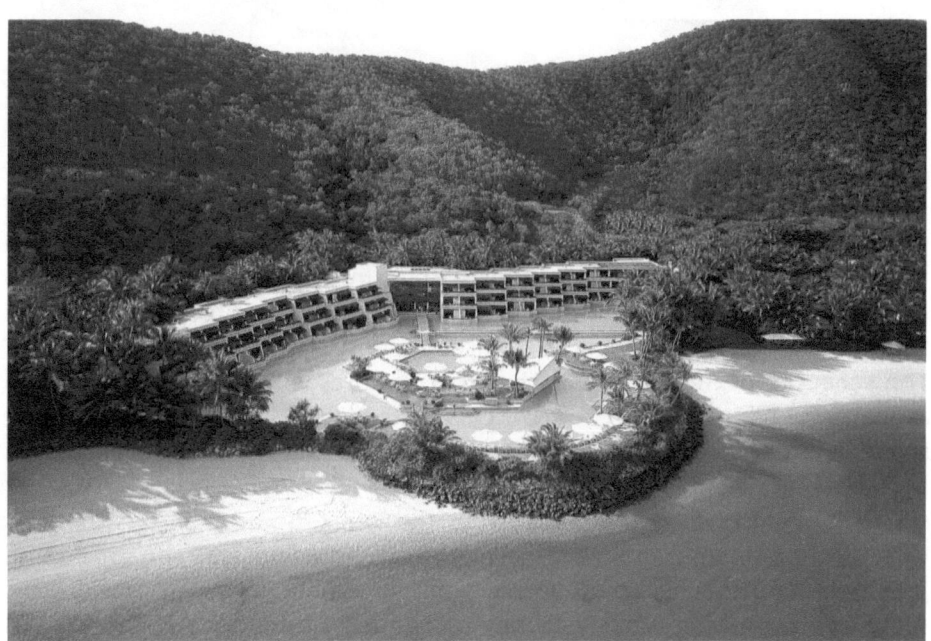

A paradise within a paradise: Hayman Islands in Australia

An Australian symposium was anticipated at least six years earlier when the Council decided to hold meetings in various areas of the world. They were cognizant of planning responsibly the locations so as not to hold meetings in excessively expensive venues or locations. Australia had many active members from the start and their involvement flourished, but it took awhile to justify the distance travel by the non-Australians. When the final decision was made, there was a three year period delay between meetings which helped to justify the additional expense.

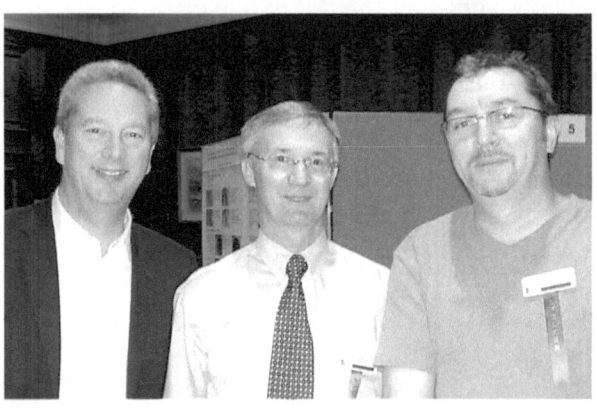

Indisputable, historical evidence that all Australian contact lens knowledge does not exist totally in Sydney: Nat Efron, Leo Carney, and Noel Brennan

Hayman Islands, located in Queensland, Australia on the Great Barrier Reef was an attractive location. Identified by the US Travel Channel as one of the ten best resorts in the world, the private island included a number of villas and rooms overlooking the tropical gardens, a lagoon, and the Coral Sea. Raymond Myers described this as being "a tropical paradise within a tropical paradise." The schedule of meetings was similar to before, with the early afternoon available for the myriad of extracurricular activities. This was the first meeting scheduled for five days where midweek—Wednesday—was left available for personal enjoyment.

One event typifies the pleasure of the week. Some members familiar with Hikaru Hamano, who was at an age which would normally be considered "retirement," knew he would be out parasailing on a particular morning. As the group sat having breakfast, they recognized Dr. Hamano in the air, and news spread among others who would likely compare their adventures to Dr. Hamano's.

Michael Lemp was President and Gerald Lowther was Program Chair for this meeting. Topics that were considered important at the time were the tears and tear interactions with the contact lens material, and infection and inflammation with contact lens wear. Keynote speakers from outside contact lenses were Linda Hazlett on *Pseudomonas aeruginosa.* Perry Binder was the session chair for "Tissue Response to Contact Lenses and Refractive Surgery: Procedure Affectivity and New Techniques for Measurement and Examinations." This session was of interest because it may have been the best example of integrating contact lenses and refractive surgery. Certain individuals known for their contact lens research—Charlene Gauthier and Jan Bergmanson—were reporting their results with refractive surgery. Barry Masters in his keynote address began to demonstrate how a confocal microscope would assist in visualizing under high magnification in vivo tissue.

8ᵗʰ Symposium—Jackson Hole, USA: September 11-15, 1995

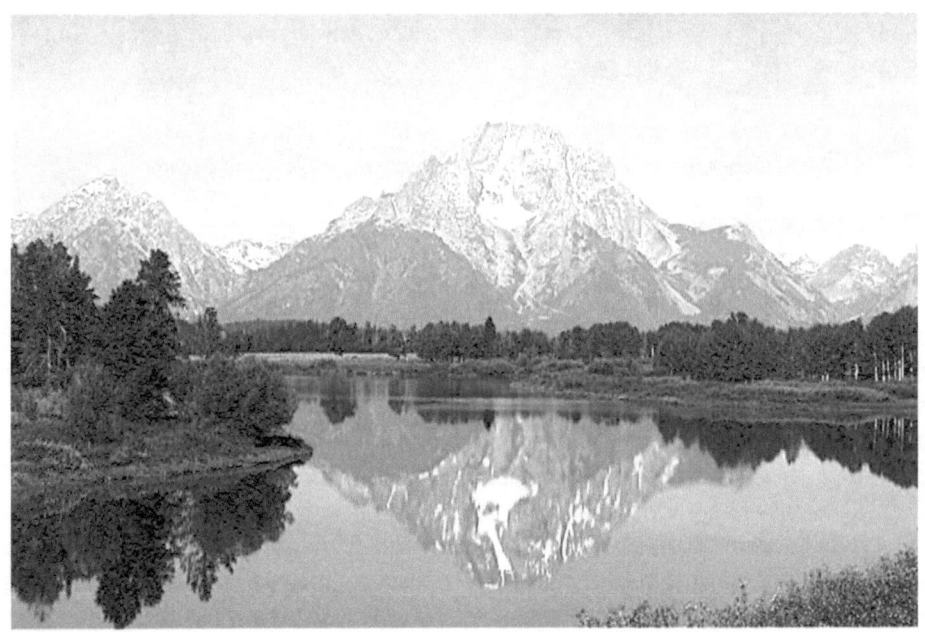

*Jackson Hole represented a picturesque glimpse and
representation of the US Rocky Mountains*

The Jackson Hole, Wyoming, venue may have been the first cooler and fall like venue since Cambridge in 1982. Located at the foot of some of the craggiest and pointed mountains of the Rocky Mountains, Jackson Hole represented a verdant and forest filled ambiance.

Gerald Lowther was President and Perry Binder the Program Chair. Inflammation and infection continued to be a major topic since past meetings and Robert Sack was the moderator of a session as was Suzanne Fleiszig. Keynote speakers included Mark Willcox and Jean Wiener-Kronish.

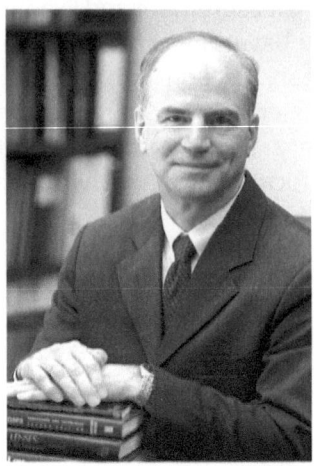

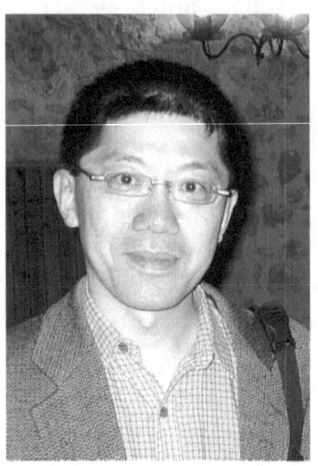

1995 President Gerald Lowther carried through with some of the most important contact lens spoilation research

Arthur Ho first came as a graduate student and became an ISCLR member in 1995

Marguerite McDonald moderated the session on refractive surgery which differed from the Hayman Symposium by almost exclusively including topics that were not connected with contact lenses. Continuous wear was a multiple session topic that included the topics of biofilm, tear flow under the lens, hypoxia, and epithelial cell changes. Visual assessment was important and this was the beginning of the consideration of spherical aberrations and wavefront optics. Council member Raymond Applegate first came as a keynote speaker in this year as did Ian Bailey who spoke on real world vision and its measurement. James Sheedy suggested that it is the performance of certain tasks which can best determine vision capability. Another keynote speaker was Mae Gordon, a biostatistician, who together with another new attendee Karla Zadnik, discussed quality of life issues that were part of the Collaborative Longitudinal Evaluation of Keratoconus.

The Jackson Hole Symposium was the first meeting that included a summary session at the end which was intended to draw broad based conclusions starting with session summaries. Although introducing this for previous meetings had been discussed, it was difficult to see how this could be inclusive considering the number of topics. But the first session on Friday morning was undertaken by Brien Holden and Perry Binder. They began to perfect the important role that ISCLR meetings performed in establishing the fundamentals of the outstanding challenges and their relationships to other areas.

9th Symposium—Florence, Italy: August 24-29, 1997

The Florence meeting was a return to Europe and the first meeting since Cambridge in 1984 which was held in a city, compared to more isolated venues. Meetings were held in a hotel with a similar schedule as the others, so that it was a difference to see other attendees at a variety of restaurants or roaming around the nearby shops.

So many of the meetings were typified by many arranged activities for the day of rest that were often typical for this area: Snorkeling and Scuba Diving at the Great Barrier Reef, White Water Rafting in Jackson Hole, Elephant rides in Phuket, and Ziplining at Whistler Mountain.

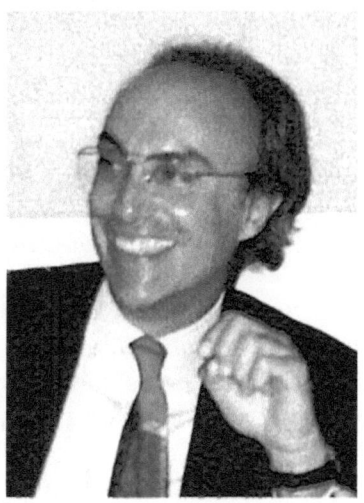
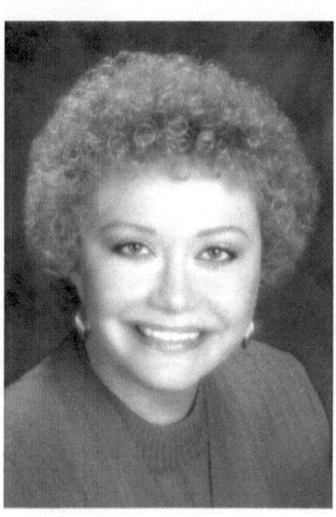

1997 President Perry Binder is a 30 year contributor with the programs and ISCLR's interprofessional character

Marguerite MacDonald succeeded Raymond Myers as VicePresident-Finance in 1997

Perry Binder was the President at this meeting and Michel Guillon was the Program Chair. This symposium began with the recognition of the forthcoming silicone hydrogels, high DK RGP's, and the subjects of chemistry, materials science, and surface properties. The first three sessions were on the new high DK hydrogel materials as well as the surfaces. Among the scientists from the manufacturers who were invited to explain the chemical basis for the new materials and properties were M K Raheja, Richard Barron, Klaus Schindlhelm and Jaergen Vogt. Among the academic scientists who had contributed extensively to past meetings were Miguel Refojo, 1986 ISCLR President and 1997 Ruben Medalist, Buddy Ratner, Brien Holden, and new contributors Clayton Radke and Jean Jacob. The appearance of new materials along with the properties which researchers and clinicians were asking for made this a very significant session. At the same time the performance of High DK RGP's were showing favorable results.

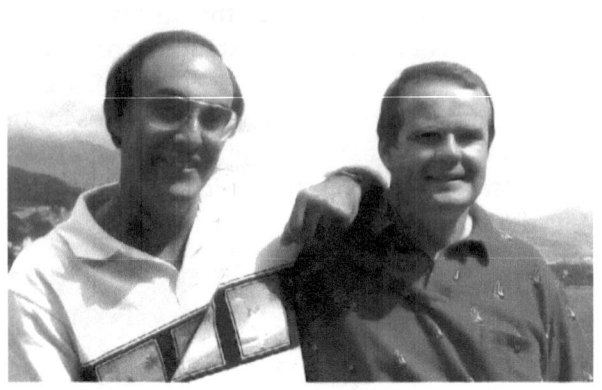

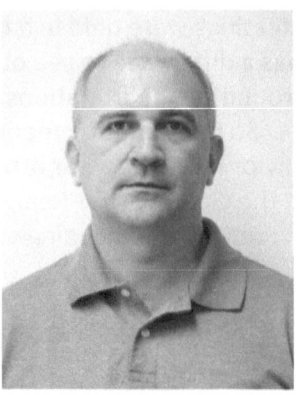

Bill Bourne and Perry Binder are good friends as well as ISCLR colleagues

Mark Willcox became a member in 1997, after being a keynote speaker the previous meeting.

The additional topic which occupied another two sessions was markers for ocular responses including inflammation and infection. Steve Wilson was the Keynote speaker presenting on cytokines and potential effects upon corneal surface in a session led by Michael Lemp and Graeme Wilson. This was followed with the last session on "Toward Continuous Wear" moderated by Michel Guillon where the summaries of earlier sessions were placed in a broader context.

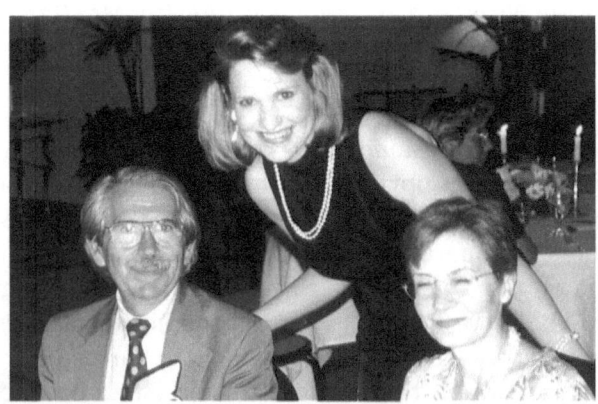

Miguel Refojo showing his Ruben Medal to Jean Jacob and his wife Svetlana

There are traditionally four group meetings during each symposium. The Executive Council meets the day before the scientific session, followed by the Council meeting on the same day. Then, Manufacturers and the Executive Council get together. At the Florence meeting the General Members Meeting became one of the more uncharacteristic and lively meetings, as reported by Secretary Deborah Sweeney. The Council passed new policies where regular members were to have two refereed published papers in a two year period and Past Presidents were to be ex officio members of the Council, according to Nathan Efron, to allow for new blood.

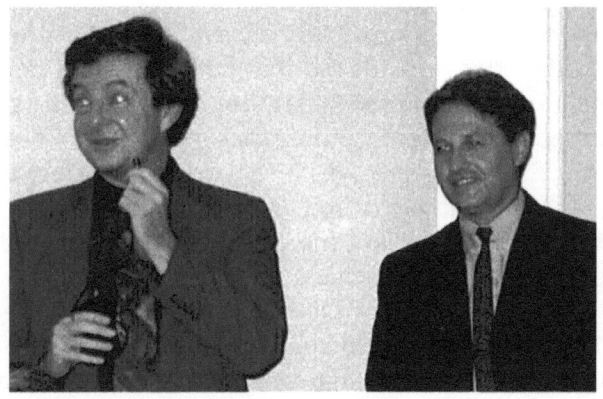

Raymond Myers and Michel Guillon report to members at the 1997 Florence Gala Dinner

Members offered a number of suggestions for the meeting. Jerry Paugh and Michael Harris pointed out that moderators needed to reinforce presentation time limits. Nathan Efron recommended an embarrassing loud buzzer which was eventually implemented. Josh Josephson felt that there should be more results and less history in presentations. Nathan Efron and Sarita Soni pointed out there needed to be more institutions represented in the graduate student selection, and Brien Holden stated that by this year's deadline 8 of the 10 submissions were from one institution. Gerald Lowther noted that they notified members and extended the deadline. The consensus was that the applications should be preselected by members from the institutions. Most membership meetings tended to be rather sedate, but in Florence certain issues and controversies would eventually make it to the Council.

10th Symposium—Phuket, Thailand: August 16-20, 1999

Phuket was one of the most historically auspicious meetings for ISCLR because of two important events. First, Otto Wichterle, ISCLR's patron and soft lens inventor, had died within the year preceding the Symposium and tributes to his legacy were presented. Second, Michel Guillon became President of the Society 21 years after he attended as a graduate student the founding meeting of the Society in London. Guillon stated in his introductory remarks, "It had been an honour for me to serve you as President following so many leaders in the field and particularly my mentor and the Society Founding President, Professor Montague Ruben."

Guillon summarized the previous 20 years of ISCLR as follows: "Looking back at these times this reminds me that during my Presidency the Society reached its majority. It was in 1978 that the concept was first developed and in 1980 the first Scientific Meeting took place at the Royal College of Surgeons in London. After its early years, which saw first the Society developing as a unique think tank in the industry and winning political battles that has made it a truly multi-disciplinary Society, the ISCLR is now mature and ready to meet the challenges of the new millennium."

Stephen Klyce was Program Chair. Ray Applegate moderated the first session and Keynoter Howard Howland focused on wave front aberrations and their significance to contact lenses and other corrective means. Holden observed that ISCLR was holding the first session in ISCLR history devoted to presbyopia. The session was led by Brien Holden and Paul Erikson on the optical and visual qualities of contact lens bifocals with Larry Thibos discussing contact lens aberrations. Also, Adrian Glasser discussed his additions to the theories of accommodation. Perry Binder discussed monovision in refractive surgery and Brien Holden presented phaco-ersatz.

A session moderated by Brian Tighe and Buddy Ratner recognized the recent availability of high Dk lenses and began considerations existing to know on lens and corneal surface compatibility including surface treatments.

11th Symposium—Sun Valley, USA: September 10-14, 2001

Sun Valley was the site of America's first ski resort. It is located in Blaine County in south, central Idaho at an elevation of 5,500 feet. The location of the symposium was at the Sun Valley Lodge which was designed in 1937 by Austrian ski instructors to portray the ambience of an Austrian resort. The nearby town of Ketchum was the residence and site of the death of American author Ernest Hemmingway. The meeting was held in the Limelight Room of Sun Valley. The Gala was in the newly built River Run Lodge at the base of Baldy Ski Mountain.

Tragically, the Sun Valley Symposium will always be characterized by 911, the attack upon the New York World Trade Center. Despite being located in Sun Valley, Idaho, Jerry Paugh has pointed out how this profoundly affected this world and even this small area. Mark Willcox recalls waking up to the dreadful news. President Steve Klyce recounts, "On the first day of the meeting, we(Marguerite McDonald and he) arose early; I was to give the opening welcome, and was anxious not to miss a lecture. However, that morning at sunrise, I called a colleague back at the lab in New Orleans with a new idea. He finished with: 'I may not start this today—a plane just crashed into the World Trade Center in New York.' Soon, Marguerite and I sat transfixed watching events exploding out of the television, too shocked and stunned to move or speak.

"So I missed my opening welcome to the ISCLR delegates, finally connecting with the meeting to learn that it had convened in spite of the extraordinary events—events more potent in their psychological impact than President Kennedy's assassination."

Even in Sun Valley the effects were direct and pointed. Steve Klyce says further, "That day, my niece and her two children lost her first responder, fireman husband. Returning home was not easy for many attendees. After the attack, airports just closed for all traffic. When they reopened, flights were just not available. But in such times of inconvenience for us, these pale by comparison to the losses suffered by the thousands who lost their lives and the further thousands of families who lost their loved ones."

Brien Holden had the dubious honor to make the first presentation on Monday, 9/11. The presentation was, "How Far Have We Come with CLs as a Form of Vision Correction Today?" Holden has performed a sustained contribution to ISCLR during these 30 years that cannot be fully recognized. Two areas in which his contributions have been enormous have been to set the stage on the issues before the group, and the second contribution at the sessions' conclusion is to draw the "big" picture from the numerous sessions. He often has done this through stimulating and colorful interaction within the group and setting the stage for future implementation.

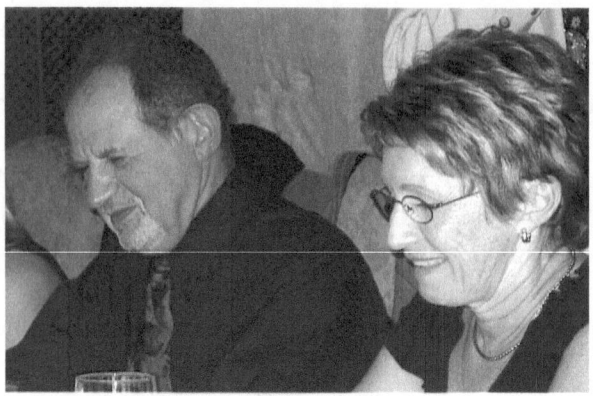

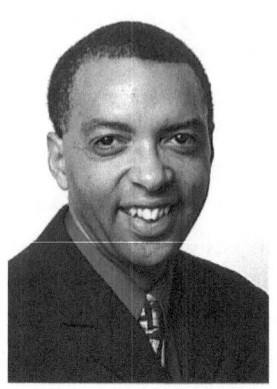

Des Fonn has held many ISCLR positions including six years as Secretary from 1993. His wife Anita contributed as de facto co-secretary

Eric Papas: graduate student in 1997 and member in 2001

Deborah Sweeney was the Program Chair for the Sun Valley Symposium. The organization of the program was divided into two parts: "Adverse Responses" and "Remaining Issues-Comfort and Vision." A significant group of keynoters presented important addresses including Michael Gilmore, Oliver Schein, Duncan Dowson, and Edwin Sarver. Sweeney as the moderator to the first session laid out the types of adverse responses that were being seen. Mark Willcox and Suzanne Fleiszig led the second session on infections and inflammation where in addition to Gilmore's presentation they initiated an extensive view of the subject of adverse complications from a clinical, basic, industrial, and applied perspective. Another session on adverse reactions was on contact lens effects and tissue reactions. A variety of areas was covered having to do with surface and bulk properties, tear exchange, and mechanical effects upon the epithelium.

The remaining four sessions on quality of life, comfort and vision were moderated by Paul Erickson, Desmond Fonn, Ian Cox, and Marguerite Mc Donald.

12th Symposium—Palma de Mallorca, Spain: September 8-12, 2003

Palma de Mallorca represented a return to Europe and a Mediterranean venue which was attractive with its island location and a warm and dry environment. The location was in large part a result of Brian Tighe's efforts and recommendation.

Deborah Sweeney assumed the Presidency at the Mallorca meeting. Among those who were not among the original charter members, Sweeney undertook extensive assignments. She has made numerous presentations and moderated panels. She worked with the Sydney group on the Proceedings from the 1988

Symposium to the present. Sweeney then assumed the Secretary position for six years in 1993 before being elected President Elect in 2001. She was also planning coordinator for the 1993 Hayman Island Symposium.

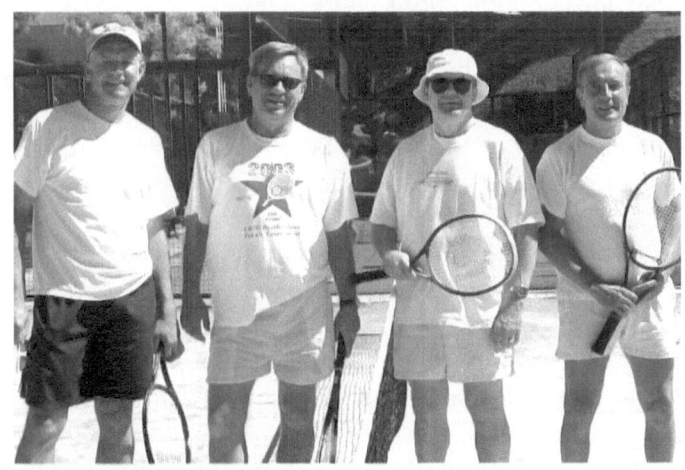

Competition extends onto the tennis court for Christopher Snyder, Jan Bergmanson, Bill Bourne, and Alan Tomlinson

Graeme Wilson was the Program Chairperson. The program theme was "Contact Lenses for Life." The first sessions revolved around myopia control introducing for the first time the work of Keynote Speaker Earl Smith speaking on emmetropization with his considerable work with primates, and Christine Wildsoet speaking on myopia control by pharmaceutical intervention or atropine. In addition, orthokeratology and its possible effects in the closed eye environment was discussed.

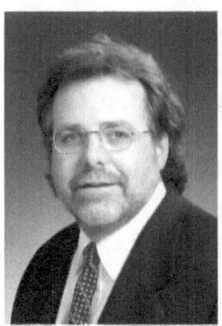

Pat Caroline became an ISCLR member at the Palma de Mallorca meeting in 2003

Additional highlights included the tear film and exchange. Clayton Radke and Anuj Chauhan made theoretical presentations on tear lens interactions and lipid spreading respectively, and Keynote Speaker Monica Berry and member Darlene Dartt looked into the function of regulation of mucins. The subjects of adverse reactions and infections were covered in two sessions moderated by Deborah Sweeney and Suzanne Fleiszig. The definition and severities of adverse reactions at the CCLRU were presented by Sweeney. Another keynote speaker was Richard O'Callaghan.

Ray Myers had not been to the Phuket or Sun Valley Symposia, and was anxious to learn what changes had occurred. He asked various individuals including Nathan Efron during an intermission to compare the last two meetings with the earlier ones. Nathan thought a minute and said of all the meetings he attends, this is his most valuable opportunity to learn and to leave with many new ideas.

There was an auspicious group of 13 members who were accepted since the last meeting which included Anuj Chauhan, Kathy Dumbleton, Barbara Fink, Gary Foulks(renewal), Michael Gilmore, Ewen King-Smith, Antonio Lopez-Alemany, Paul Murphy, Jason Nichols, Kelly Nichols, Oliver Schein, Michelle Senchyna, and Graeme Young.

13th Symposium—Coolum Beach, Australia: August 15-19, 2005

The Coolum Beach Symposium was a second Symposium for Australia, this time to a coastal vacation area south of Brisbane and one of the great surfing areas in the country. The President was Graeme Wilson and the Program Chair was Desmond Fonn. In his opening remarks, Wilson gave credit to those who made the Society into what it is today.

> *Much of the success of ISCLR comes from the effort and dedication of its members. In addition, the invited students bring a fresh enthusiasm to contact lens research, and it is a great privilege to be able to support the development of tomorrow's leaders in this field. Industry representatives are an integral part of ISCLR and we are indebted to their continued support and also their active personal participation at each meeting. All in all, ISCLR is a remarkable mix of industry, university, youth, experience, professions and nationalities. Long may it continue.*

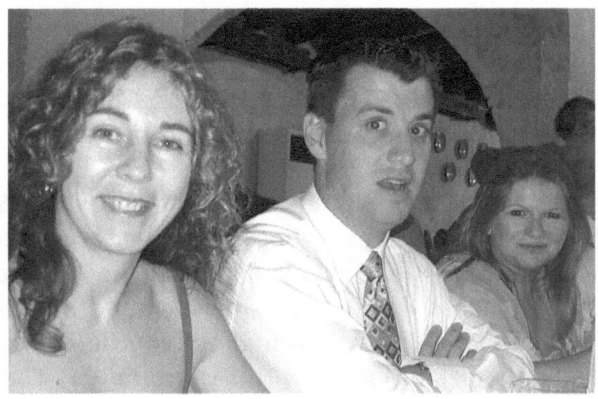

*President Suzanne Fleiszig sits with Philip Morgan, ISCLR
Secretary since 1995; with his wife Sarah*

The Coolum meeting was striking in that the first four topics were contact lens complications divided into epidemiology, etiology and pathogenesis of complications, other adverse reactions, and technology/techniques for measurement. In the first session topic for epidemiology, two new contributors were John Dart and Oliver Schein with member Fiona Stapleton. In the etiology and pathogenesis session two new contributors were Michael Gilmore, co-moderator with Suzanne Fleiszig and Gerald Pier. The next four topics were variations of considerations of contact lens and ocular surfaces with measurement techniques. New keynote speakers were Jay McLaren and Richard O'Callaghan.

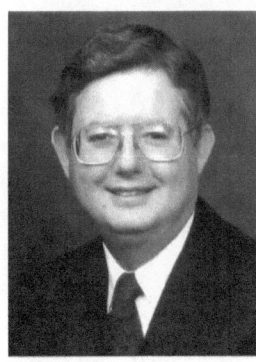

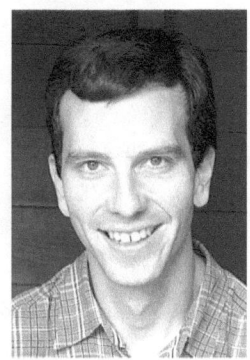

Dwight Cavanagh became vice president in Coolum Beach having had other roles since 1990

James Wolffsohn became a member in 2001 having come earlier as a graduate student

Two new approaches also used in 2007 were introduced in Coolum Beach. The first was a session for graduate students and the introduction of graduate student posters. Richard Hill spearheaded this as well as earlier efforts to make the graduate student efforts an integral part of ISCLR.

There was discussion at the Council meeting about the ISCLR becoming more involved in forming interest groups whenever an would benefit from group consensus such as the previous efforts at the Montreal symposium where standardized lenses were used to make cross comparisons of oxygen measurement techniques. An additional activity began last meeting for developing grading scales called the CHASM group. Des Fonn in particular wanted this effort to expand, to which Raymond Applegate felt this would also be useful in wave aberration areas.

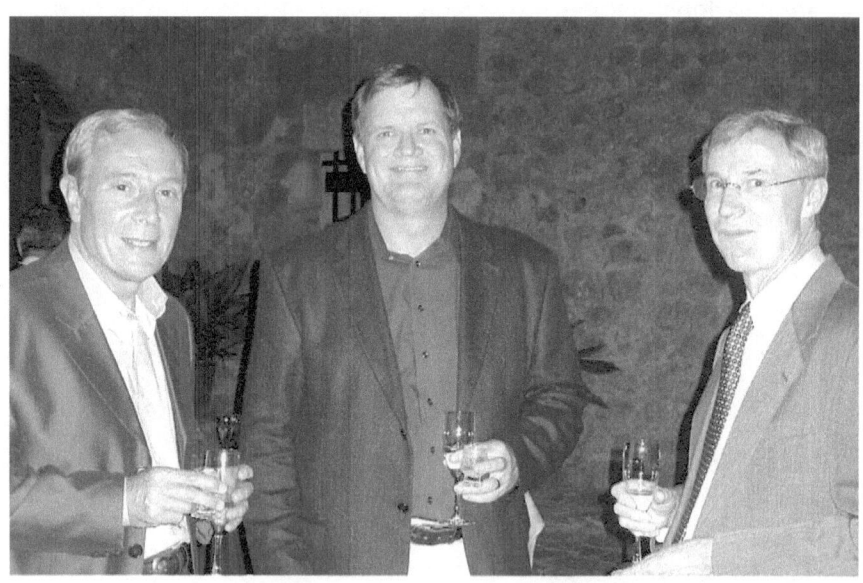

Longtime members representing three continents:
Alan Tomlinson, Joseph Benjamin, and Leo Carney

14th Symposium—Whistler Mountain, Canada: August 13-17, 2007

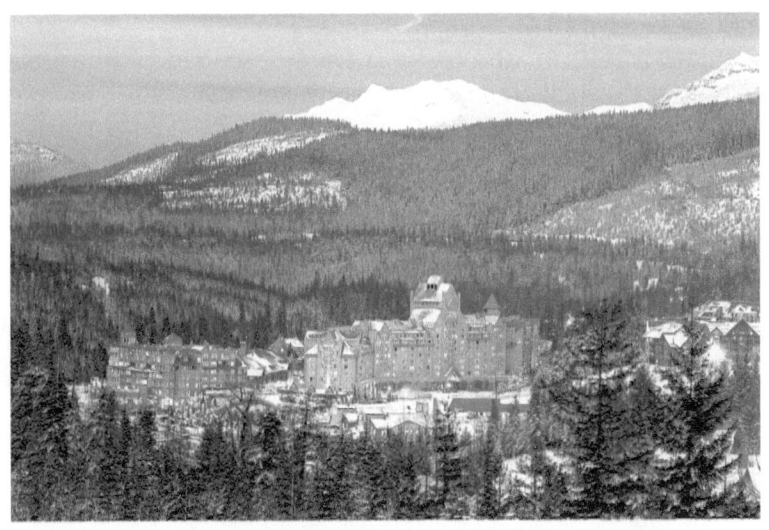

*Chateau Whistler Hotel near Vancouver, BC, was the
2007 Symposium location*

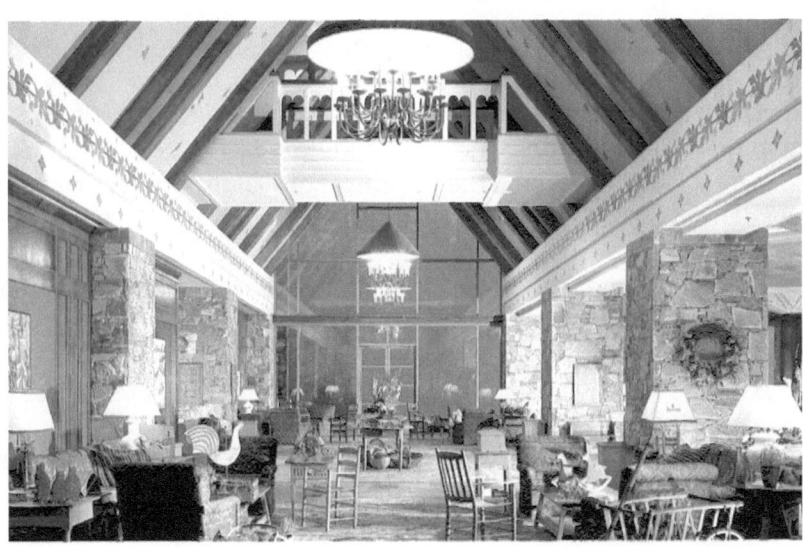

*The lobby of the Chateau Whistler Lodge was a central
meeting place with the restaurant off to the right*

The 14th Symposium was held in the appealing Chateau Whistler Hotel, a lodge at the base of Whistler Mountain north of Vancouver, British Columbia, and was recommended by President Desmond Fonn. Suzanne Fleiszig was the Program Chair for this 15 session symposium.

The major subjects for the sessions were described by three questions, and six invited speakers were involved to give Keynote addresses.

- How do we solve infections and inflammations (6 sessions)

    ○ Eric Perlman—Fusarium keratitis
    ○ Kermit Carraway—Mucous
    ○ Robert Hancock—Antimicrobial peptides

- How do we resolve discomfort and dryness (3 sessions)

    ○ Stephen Pflugfelder—Dry eye and ocular surface inflammation
    ○ Richard Linhardt—Synthetic mucin analogues

- How do we improve vision

    ○ Jason Marsack—Wavefront contact lens considerations

The summary and last session—co-moderated by Brien Holden, Suzanne Fleiszig and Dwight Cavanagh—was an example of how the program was organized to handle a number of individual topics but to devote most of the time for interaction. The questions below were the condensation of the important questions from discussions, and the responses of a large number of individuals were condensed by the Proceedings authors into one or more sentences.

- *What are the greatest current challenges remaining to the understanding of pathogenesis and prevention of lens-related microbial keratitis (MK)?*
- *Is there a role of lens-induced or solution-related damage to the surface corneal epithelium that increases MK?*
- *What can past and ongoing Clinical Epidemiological Studies tell us about how to identify and prevent lens-related MK?*
- *What specific areas are "ripe" for future studies to decrease MK rates?*
- *What is the role of contact lens-related care solution in producing "cornea staining" of and/or "loss" of surface cells and does this increase risk for MK?*

- *What are new technology or new ideas that we need to work on before the next meeting?*
- *Audience Poll: Does manufacturer surface "coating" of lenses predict "comfort" in the eye?*
- *Where are we with current optical refractive instruments, technology and correction?*
- *What is the current present and future of orthokeratology?*
- *Is there a clinical role for artificial Corneal Onlays-Inlays in refractive correction?*
- *What are the most important needs for the next 2 years?*

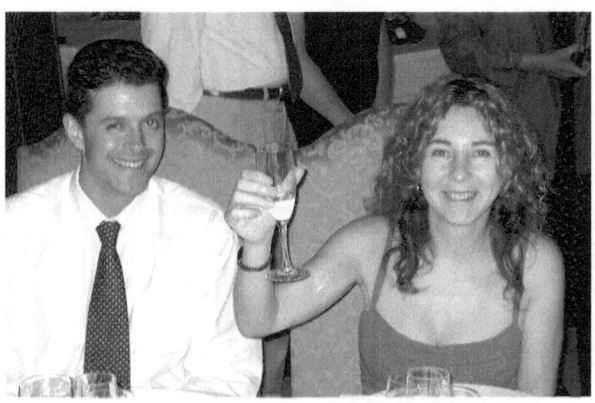

President(2009) Suzanne Fleiszig and her husband, member David Evans

Postcript

Future of ISCLR

The Origins and Ethos of the ISCLR
by Brien A Holden

Let me say firstly Ray Myers has provided a wonderful and as far as I can tell, accurate chronicling of the origins, activities and progress of the ISCLR. Ray was the instigator of the Society even though he was seeking an organisation with a different remit - an international federation of contact lens societies and associations. When I arrived in that Moorfields Board room in 1978, after experiencing the non-stop 72 hour mid-summer celebration with Antti Vannas on his beloved island Finnholm, it struck me that the politics and complications of what Ray was, nobly, trying to do, would be a nightmare. At that time relations between ophthalmology and optometry had dimensions that would challenge the United Nations Secretary General. And it was only pure and unadulterated souls like Monty Ruben, and later the almost as pure souls of Mike Lemp, Perry Binder, Steve Klyce, Marguerite Mc Donald, and Dwight Cavanagh who would dare challenge the trade union norms and put their heads on the chopping block of scientific co-mingling.

It seemed to me that what we needed in 1978 to advance contact lenses (and I think still do), was knowledge and understanding. We had had a number of meltdowns and failures in the industry such as extended wear infections and poorly performing bifocals and we really needed to dig deeper into mechanisms and scientific understanding.

Monty was at first a little dubious but quickly warmed to the idea and developed an ethos around the Society of the pursuit of rigorous science, truth, and an open, commercial-free exchange of knowledge. Under his stewardship and those after him, the ISCLR grew into the wonderful think-tank that it has been for 30 years. In this role the ISCLR provided an opportunity for frank and open communication on the latest research and ideas from the clinicians and researchers, intermingled with the input from outstanding 'outsiders' from the world of science; people who often became insiders and vital on-going ISCLR contributors and occasionally, our colleagues in industry (at least in the hushed hallways).

Monty was a great first President as he had that dignity, scientific integrity and commitment to honesty that ensured that the society would fulfil its destiny.

Ray asked me to address a number of questions in this reflective piece on my personal perspective of the ISCLR. So, as was the norm in the early days, I always do what Ray asks, because I have rarely met a person whose selfless dedication to keeping an idea and an organisation on a righteous path exceeded that of the great Ray Myers.

What has ISCLR contributed to the research field?

The ISCLR contributed an opportunity for all 'categories' of researchers the young, the older, the basic, the clinical, the industry, the specialist; to meet and talk in closed session about the issues of the day and the future research needed to understand how to improve the contact lens experience for the tens of millions of wearers of these very useful devices. The ISCLR provided an opportunity to hear Irv Fatt rip the sloppy heart out of an unscientific piece of work or Frank Holly bring great knowledge to bear on the biophysics of surfaces or Miguel Refojo place a scientific construct around polymers and their behaviour. It provided an opportunity for the clinical researchers to stand up to the excessively esoteric basic scientists now and again re-grounding their frameworks in the clinical realities. It encouraged, at their own risk, the 'up and coming' to challenge the dogma of the presumed 'down and going'. It provided an opportunity for industry researchers and other professionals to sit and listen to the back and forth on the hot topics of the day.

But most of all, the ISCLR provided an opportunity to think about the challenges and the concepts in a collegial environment with the best researchers the ISCLR could muster, funded by an appreciative industry.

Where will ISCLR be in the long term future?

The industry seems to have been stagnant at 100 million or so wearers worldwide for the last 10 years. Ten to fifteen percent drop out of lenses each year due to discomfort and adverse event – at rates that are too high and have not changed in years, except perhaps with daily disposables. ISCLR is still sorely needed. In fact it needs to lift its game as the contact lens industry's innovation think tank to tackle the more difficult issues that are left.

The ISCLR must continue thru its Executive and Councillors to seek the best of the young blood through student sponsorships and exposure to the meeting and encourage and foster their participation. The ISCLR has never really been successful at getting industry scientists to participate (with a few notable exceptions) in the forums, but getting their input on the issues ISCLR needs to be tackling is vital.

Through the Executive and Meetings process and especially through the Chairs of the Scientific Sessions, the ISCLR must bring in new scientists working in related fields, excite them and educate them about the challenges we face and get them involved not only with the Society but its researchers and aspirations.

What prior characteristics ensure its continuation?

Freedom for participants to speak freely of their cutting edge work without fear of the work being "stolen" or quoted, in an atmosphere of mutual scientific enquiry on key issues.

Spirited debate about the work presented so that industry can gain access not only to the network of researchers but also to their thoughts and summary sessions for wrapping up issues and new potential directions.

Appendices

Appendix 1

Symposia of the International Society for Contact Lens Research

1st Symposium—London, England—1980
2nd Symposium—Montreal, Canada—1982
3rd Symposium—Cambridge, England—1984
4th Symposium—S'Agaro, Spain—1986
5th Symposium—Kauai, USA—1988
6th Symposium—Monte Carlo, Monaco—1990
7th Symposium—Hayman Island, Australia—1993
8th Symposium—Jackson Hole, USA—1995
9th Symposium—Florence, Italy—1997
10th Symposium—Phuket, Thailand—1999
11th Symposium—Sun Valley, USA—2001
12th Symposium—Palma de Mallorca, Spain—2003
13th Symposium—Coolum Beach, Australia-2005
14th Symposium—Whistler Mountain, Canada-2007
15th Symposium—Creta Maris, Crete—2009

Appendix 2

Founding Council Members

OFFICERS

MONTAGUE RUBEN, PRESIDENT
BRIEN HOLDEN, PRESIDENT-ELECT
RICHARD HILL, VICE PRESIDENT

MICHAEL LEMP, VICE PRESIDENT
MIGUEL REFOJO, VICE PRESIDENT
RAYMOND I. MYERS, SECRETARY
TREASURER

LEO CARNEY
WULF EHRICH
IRVING FATT
HIKARU HAMANO
RICHARD M. HILL
FRANK J. HOLLY
RICHARD I. KEATES
ROBERT A. KOETTING
DONALD KORB
MICHAIL M. KRASNOV
JOHN LARKE
MICHAEL LEMP
GERALD E. LOWTHER

IAN MACKIE
ROBERT B. MANDELL
DAVID MAURICE
SAIICHI MISHIMA
KENNETH POLSE
MAURICE POSTER
MIGUEL F. REFOJO
HANS-WALTER ROTH
JANET STONE
PAUL F. WHITE
OTTO WICHTERLE
PETER WRIGHT

Appendix 3

Charter Members

International Society for Contact Lens Research

Nur	Ahmed	UK
James	Aquavella	USA
Philip	Baronet	France
Perry	Binder	USA
Roger	Buckley	UK
Murchison	Callendar	Canada
Leo	Carney	Australia
Jennifer	Chaston	UK
Barry	Collin	Australia
Donald	Doughman	USA
W	Ehrich	Germany
Daniel	Epstein	Switzerland
Stuart	Eriksen	USA
Joan	Exford Korb	USA
Peter	Fanti	Germany
Irving	Fatt	USA
Victor	Finnemore	USA
Guenter	Forst	Germany
Gary	Foulks	USA
Leon	Garner	New Zealand

Michel	**Guillon**	**UK**
Hikaru	**Hamano**	**Japan**
Michael	**Harris**	**USA**
Antonio	**Henriquez**	**Spain**
Richard	**Hill**	**USA**
Nizar	**Hirji**	**UK**
Brien	**Holden**	**Australia**
Frank	**Holly**	**USA**
Joshua	**Josephson**	**Canada**
Richard	**Keates**	**USA**
Angela	**Kempster**	**UK**
Jonathan	**Kersley**	**UK**
Yoshizo	**Kikkawa**	**Japan**
Robert	**Koetting**	**USA**
Donald	**Korb**	**USA**
M.	**Krasnov**	**Russia**
Francois	**Kreiss-Gosselin**	**France**
Lubomir	**Krejci**	**Czechoslovakia**
David	**Lamberts**	**USA**
John	**Larke**	**UK**
Michael	**Lemp**	**USA**
Richard	**Lindstrom**	**USA**
David	**Lobascher**	**UK**
D.F.C.	**Loran**	**UK**
Gerald	**Lowther**	**USA**
Donald	**MacKeen**	**USA**
Ian	**Mackie**	**UK**
Robert	**Mandell**	**USA**
Barry	**Masters**	**USA**
David	**Maurice**	**USA**
Charles	**McMonnies**	**Australia**
George	**Mertz**	**USA**
David	**Miller**	**USA**
Michel	**Millodot**	**UK**

Judith	**Morris**	**UK**
Raymond	**Myers**	**USA**
Sven Erik	**Nilsson**	**Sweden**
Richard	**Pearson**	**UK**
Tomas	**Pfortner**	**Argentina**
Anthony	**Phillips**	**Australia**
Kenneth	**Polse**	**USA**
Michael	**Port**	**UK**
Maurice	**Poster**	**USA**
Buddy	**Ratner**	**USA**
Miguel	**Refojo**	**USA**
Roy	**Rengstorff**	**USA**
Pierre	**Rocher**	**France**
Enrico	**Romani**	**Italy**
HW	**Roth**	**Germany**
Montague	**Ruben**	**UK**
William	**Sammons**	**UK**
Morton	**Sarver**	**USA**
Michael	**Sheridan**	**UK**
Sarita	**Soni**	**USA**
Thomas	**Spring**	**Australia**
Walter	**Stark**	**USA**
Janet	**Stone**	**UK**
Ranier	**Sundmacher**	**Germany**
Alan	**Tomlinson**	**UK**
Antti	**Vannas**	**Finland**
Sheldon	**Wechsler**	**USA**
Paul	**White**	**USA**
Otto	**Wichterle**	**Czechoslovakia**
Louis	**Wilson**	**USA**
Geoffrey	**Woodward**	**UK**
Peter	**Wright**	**UK**
Steven	**Zantos**	**Australia**

Appendix 4

ISCLR PRESIDENTS

Dwight Cavanagh 2009-2011
Suzanne Fleiszig 2007-2009
Desmond Fonn 2005-2007
Graeme Wilson 2003-2005
Deborah Sweeney 2001-2003
Stephen Klyce 1999-2001
Michel Guillon 1997-1999
Perry Binder 1995-1997
Gerald Lowther 1993-1995
Michael Lemp 1990-1993
Richard Hill 1988-1990
Kenneth Polse 1986-1988
Miguel Refojo 1984-1986
Brien Holden 1982-1984
Montague Ruben—1980-1982 Founding President

Appendix 5

Ruben Metal WINNERS

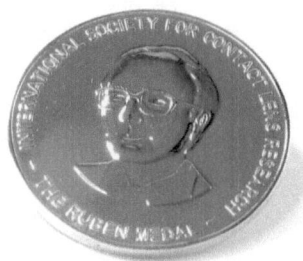

The Ruben Metal has recognized the sustained contributions of a number of ISCLR's important researchers

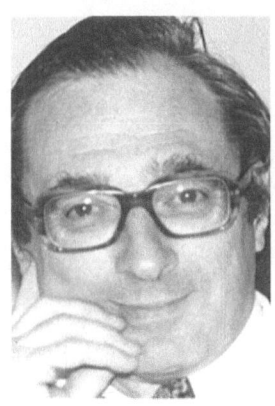

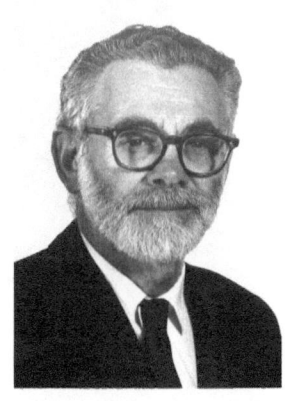

Montague Ruben; Co-founder(1984)   *Irvin Fatt(1988)*

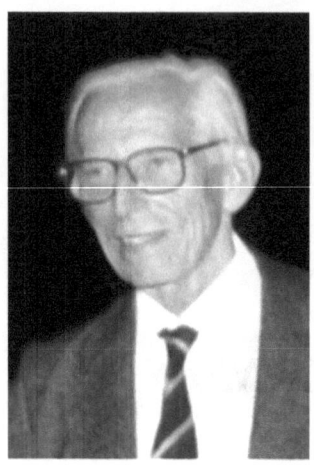

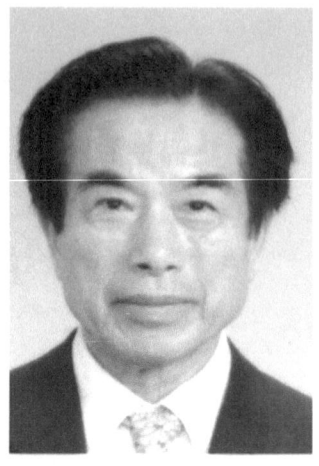

Otto Witcherle(1990)   *Hikaru Hamano(1993)*

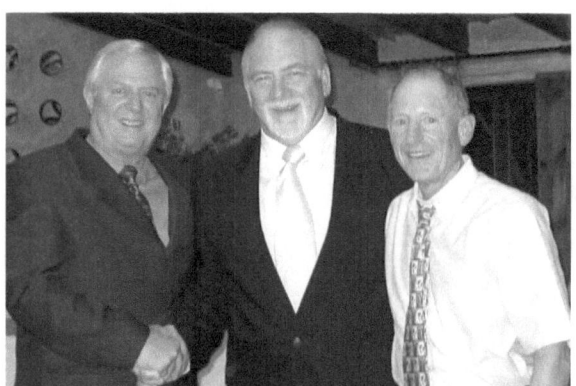

Ruben Medallists Stephen Klyce(2003), Brien Holden(1986),
and Kenneth Polse(2001)

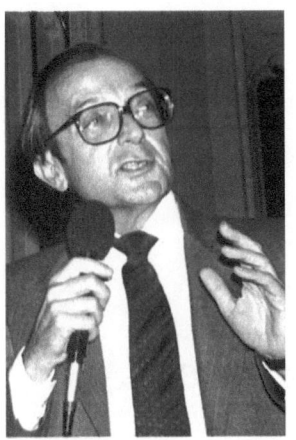

Donald Korb(1995)

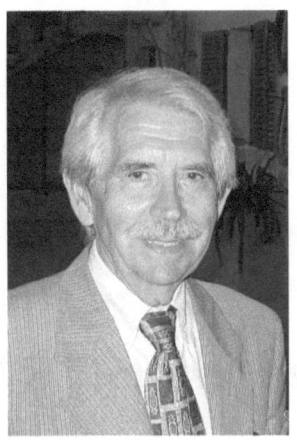

Miguel Refojo(1997)

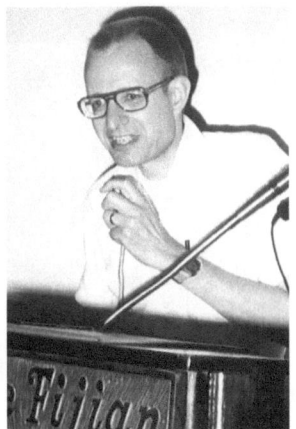

Richard Hill(1999)

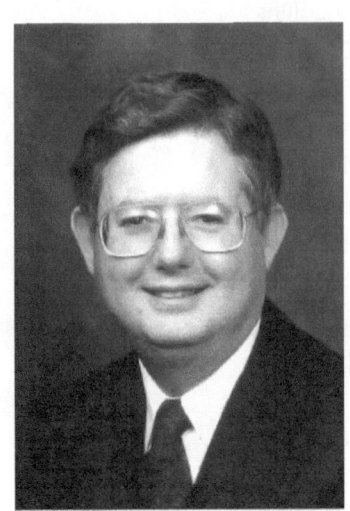

Dwight Cavanagh(2005)

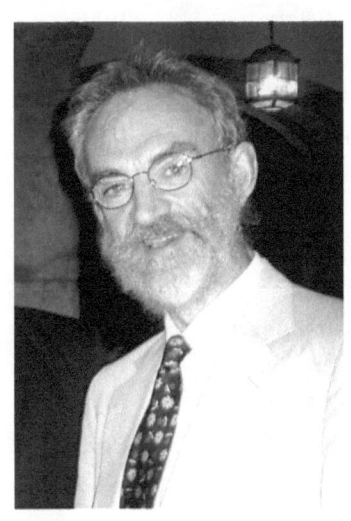

Graeme Wilson(2007)

Appendix 6

Past & Current ISCLR Members

Murali K Aasuri		Jennifer Chaston	1980-85
Nur Ahmed	1980-91	Anuj Chauhan	2003-
Raymond Applegate	1997-	Pauline Cho	2005-
James Aquavella	1980-1991	Leena Way Chu	1986-94
Arthur Back	2001-	Chantal	2007-
Howard Backman	1986-96	Coles-Brennan	
Philip Baronet	1980-1994	Michael Collins	1995-2002
Joseph Barr	1986-	Barry Collins	
Brian Barsky	2003-2006	Ian Cox	1995-
Jules Baum	2001-2006	Anthony Cullen	1990-1998
William J. Benjamin	1986-	Darlene Dartt	2001-
Jan Bergmanson	1984-	Noel Dilly	2001-2004
Perry Binder	1980-	Marshall Doane	1986-
Joseph Bonano	1993-94	Peter Donshik	1995-2004
Irving Borish	1988-	Donald Doughman	1980-1984
William J Bourne	1988-	Kathy Dumbleton	2003-
Noel Brennan	1986-	Michael Dunn	1995-
Adrian Bruce	1993-2002	Nathan Efron	1984-
Roger Buckley	1982-2004	Donald Egan	1988-
Barbara Caffery	1986-	W Ehrich	1980-84
Murchison Callendar	1980-2004	Daniel Epstein	1980-
Leo Carney	1980-	Paul Erickson	1993-
Patrick Caroline	1993-	Stuart Eriksen	1980-1989
H. Dwight Cavanagh	1988-	David Evans	2001-

Joan Exford	1982-2006	Jonathon Kersley	1980-1994
Peter Fanti	1980-	Yoshizo Kikkawa	1980-1987
Lindsy Farris	1995-2002	Ewen King-Smith	2003-
Irving Fatt	1980-2000	Stanley A. Klein	2001-2004
Barbara Fink	2003-	Stephen Klyce	1988-
Victor Finnemore	1982-2004	Robert Koetting	1980-
Suzanne Fleiszig	1995-	Donald Korb	1980-2006
Desmond Fonn	1984-	Gregory Kracher	1986-1992
Guenter Forst	1980-1994	M. Krasnov	1980-1987
Gary Foulks	1980-	R Krefman	
Leon Garner	1980-1989	Fracois Kreiss-Gosselin	1982-1996
Qian Garrett	2007-	Lubomir Krejci	1982-1985
Charlene Gauthier	1995-	J Kress	1986-1990
Michael Gilmore	2003-	Stephen Kwok	1990-1996
Hans J. Grieser	2001-2	Patrick Ladage	2005-2006
Michel Guillon	1980-	Donna LaHood	1993-2006
Hikaru Hamano	1980-	Carol Lakkis	2001-
Michael Harris	1982-	David Lamberts	1980-1994
Dean Hart	1998-	John Larke	1980-1994
Jack Hartstein	1990-1994	Robert Lavker	2007-
Antonio Henriquez	1980-	Michael Lemp	1980-
Richard Hill	1980-	Brian Levy	1988-
Nizar Hirji	1980-1989	Meng Lin	2005-
Arthur Ho	1995-	Richard Lindstrom	1982-1989
Brien Holden	1980-	Andrew Lloyd	2001-2006
Frank Holly	1980-1994	David Lobascher	1980-1985
Joseph Huff	1993-1998	Antonio	2003-
Emma Hume	2001-	Lopez-Alemany	
Jean Jacob	1997-	D.F.C. Loran	1980-1985
Isabelle Jalbert	2005-	Russel Lowe	2001-
Lyndon W. Jones	2001-	Gerald Lowther	1980-
Joshua Josephson	1980-	Donald MacKeen	1980-1983
Richard Keates	1980-1987	Ian Mackie	1980-9 &
Lisa Keay	2007-		1995-2004
Angela Kempster	1980-1985	Nayouki Maeda	2001-2006
Yshino Kenichi	1999-2000	Carole Maldonado	2005-
		Florence Malet	1995-1996

Name	Years	Name	Years
Robert Mandell	1980-1991	Anthony Phillips	1980-2000
Marechal-Courtois	1990-1996	Donald Pitts	1986-1992
Kajita Masayoshi	2007-	Kenneth Polse	1980-
Barry Masters	1982-1996	Michael Port	1980-86 &
William Mathers	1990-2004		1995-02
David Maurice	1980-1985	Maurice Poster	1980-2002
Alison McDermott	2007-	Clayton J Radke	2001-
Marguerite McDonald	1995-	G. Nag Rao	1995-2004
Timothy McMahon	1995-	Buddy Ratner	1980-
Charles McMonnies	1980-	Miguel Refojo	1980-
Nancy A. McNamara	2001-	Roy Rengstorff	1980-1996
George Mertz	1980-	Pierre Rocher	1980-
David Miller	1980-1985	Enrico Romani	1982-1985
William Miller	2007-	Perry Rosenthal	1990-
Michelle Millodot	1982-1987	HW Roth	1980-1989
Dorla Mirjeovsky	1995-1998	Montague Ruben	1980-
S. Mishima	1980-1981	Robert Sack	1997-2002
Frank Molock	2007-	William Sammons	1980-1989
Philip B. Morgan	1993-	Padmaja R.	1999-
Carol Morris	1997-	Sankaridurg	
Judith Morris	1980-	Morton Sarver	1980-
John Mountford	2005-	Oliver Schein	2003-
Eric Pealman	2007-	Cristina Schnider	1995-
Paul Murphy	2003-	Michelle Senchyna	2003-2006
Raymond Myers	1980-	Savitri Sharma	2003-2006
Jason Nichols	2003-	Michael Sheridan	1980-1087
Kelly Nichols	2003-	Trefford Simpson	2001-
Sven Erik Nilsson	1980-	Earl Smith	2005-
Clare O'Donnell	2007-	Christopher Snyder	1995-
Daniel O'Leary	1986-2000	Gabor A. Somorjai	2001-
Melvin O'Neal	1996-2001	Sarita Soni	1982-2006
Eric Papas	2001-	Thomas Spring	1980-1992
Sudi Patel	1997-2006	Fiona Stapleton	1995-
Jerry Paugh	1995-	Walter Stark	1980-1994
Richard Pearson	1980-	Ralph Stone	2007-
Gerald Pier	2007-	Janet Stone	1980-
Tomas Pfortner	1980-1987	Rainer Sundmacher	1980-1985

Helen Swarbrick	1995-		Louis Wilson	1980-1996
Deborah Sweeney	1990-		Lynn Winterton	2007-
Loretta Szczotka-Flynn	2005-		James Wolffsohn	2005-
Brian Tighe	1984-		Craig Woods	2001-
Alan Tomlinson	1980-		Geoffrey Woodward	1980-1998
Ramesh Tripathi	1995-1996		Peter Wright	1980-1996
Antti Vannas	1982-2006		Stan Yamane	1988-1994
Jay Wang	2005-		Kenichi Yoshino	2003-2004
Sheldon Wechsler	1980-1996		Graeme Young	2003-2006
Paul White	1980-1987		Karla Zadnik	1995-2002
Otto Wichterle	1980-		Steven Zantos	1982-2000
Mark Willcox	1997-		Barry Zhang-Weissman	1988-
Graeme Wilson	1986-			
Steven Wilson	1995-2002			

Appendix 7

Keynote Speakers

(ISCLR members designated by an *)

1988	Mathea Allensmith	Boston, Massachusetts	Bacterial adherance to contact lenses
1995	Raymond Applegate*	Houston, Texas	Using aberration structures to evaluate corneal optical function
1995	Ian Bailey	Berkeley, California	Assessment of real work vision-visual resolution: Assessment of real work vision-quality of subjective vision
2003	Carlos Belmonte	San Juan de Alicante, Spain	The sensory basis for ocular comfort/discomfort
1986	Carlos Belmonte	San Juan de Alicante, Spain	Neural response to mechanical stimulation of the cornea
2003	Monica Berry	Bristol, United Kingdom	Ocular mucins and contact lens wear
1986	Perry Binder*	San Diego, California	Overview of refractive surger
2003	Joseph Bonano*	Bloomington, Indiana	Oxygen in contact lens wear—2003
1999	William Bourne*	Rochester, Minnesota	Recent methods of assessing corneal functions
2007	Kermit Carroway	Miami, Florida	Mucins of the ocular surface
2003	Dwight Cavanagh*	Washington D.C.	Corneal Epithelial Homeostasis in Contact Lens Wear

1990	Dwight Cavanagh*	Washington D.C.	Confocal Microscopy: A New Imaging Paradigm
1990	John Chandler	Seattle, Washington	Contact Lens-Related Ocular Immunology
2001	Anuj Chauhan*	Gainesville, Florida	Dynamic settling of a soft lens
1995	William Costerton	Los Angeles, California	Biofilm surface interaction
2005	John Dart	London, United Kingdom	Epidemiology of contact lens related keratitits-A perspective and results from a UK case control study
2003	Darlene Dartt*	Boston, Massachusetts	The ocular surface epithelial basis for ocular comfort/discomfort
1999	Darlene Dartt*	Boston, Massachusetts	Regulation of tear secretion
1993	Noel Dilly*	Tooting, United Kingdom	Recent advances in tear film ultrastructure
2001	Duncan Dowson	Oklahoma City, US	Biotribology at other body sites
1984	Irvin Fatt*	Berkeley, California	Physical properties of materials
1993	Suzanne Fleiszig*	Boston, Massachusetts	The pathogenesis of contact lens-related infectious keratitis
1999	Suzanne Fleiszig*	Berkeley, California	The pathogenesis of contact lens-related infections
1982	Guenter Forst*	Berlin, Germany	Tear film structure and function
1984	Michael Freeman	Clwyd, United Kingdom	Retinal image and chromatic aberration
2001	Michael Gilmore*	Boston, Massachusetts	Bugs, cornea, and immunology
1995	Mae Gordon	St. Louis, Missouri	Contact Lenses and the Quality of Life
1993	John Grievenkamp	Tucson, Airizona	Optical acuity predictions using ray tracing models
2007	Robert Hancock	Vancouver, Canada	Antimicrobial peptides and their effects on microbes and the immune system
1999	Daniel Harvitt	Berkeley, California	Physiology and Pathophysiology
1993	Linda Hazlett	Detroit, Michigan	Pseudomonas aeruginosa corneal infections: adhesion, inflammation and keratitis
1984	Brien Holden*	Sydney, Australia	The Endothelium

1982	Brien Holden*	Sydney, Australia	Role and effect of lens movement
1982	Frank Holly*	Lubbock, Texas	Interaction of Tears and Lens in Safe Extended Wear
1999	Howard C. Howland	Ithaca, New York	Principles and assumptions of wavefront sensing
1999	Stanley Klein	Berkeley, California	What can corneal mapping tell us about lens motion and mechanical behaviors?
1990	Donald Korb*	Boston, Massachusetts	Lens Design and Performance
2005	Robert Lavker*	Chicago, Illinois	What's new in palpebral epithelium
1990	Richard Lembach	Columbus, Ohio	The Future of Contact Lens Research
1986	Drahoslav Lim	Las Vegas, Nevada	Mechanisms of deposit formation
2007	Richard Linhart	Troy, New York	Synthetic mucin analogs for surface modification
1982	Robert Mandell*	Berkeley, California	Extended wear of contact lenses
2007	Jason Marsack	Houston, Texas	The emergence of wavefront guided contact lenses
1993	Barry Masters*	Bethesda, Maryland	Current and future potential of confocal microscopy in contact lens and refractive surgery research
1984	Barry Masters*	Bethesda, Maryland	The Epithelium
2003	Jay McLaren	Rochester, Minnesota	Challenges in measuring corneal thickness and keratocyte density
1984	Sven Eric Nilsson*	Linköping, Sweden	Acids, alkalis and toxins acting on contact lenses
2003	Richard O'Callaghan	Jackson, Mississippi	Experimental Staphylococcus Keratitis; Host defense and pathogenesis
2007	Eric Pearlman*	Cleveland, Ohio	Fusarium Keratitis
2007	Steve Plugfelder	Houston, Texas	Dry eye and ocular surface inflammation, comparisons with contact lens wear
2005	Gerald Pier*	Boston, Massachusetts	Pseudomonas aeruginosa and corneal infection
1990	Kenneth Polse*	Berkeley, California	Lens/Cornea Interactions

1995	Kenneth Polse*	Berkeley, California	Ocular responses to extended wear: what we know, and we don't know
2003	Clayton Radke*	Berkeley, California	Interaction of Tears and Lens in Safe Extended Wear
1999	Clayton Radke*	Berkeley, California	Tear Exchange under a Soft Contact Lens: An Overview
1993	Buddy Ratner*	Seattle, Washington	Thoughts on contact lens biointeraction: protein or no protein
1982	Miguel Refojo*	Boston, Massachusetts	Gas permeable hard lenses containing silicone
1999	Robert Sack*	New York, New York	The role of proteases and anti-proteases in inflammation
2001	Edwin Sarver	San Antonio, TX	Higher order aberrations in the general population and the visual benefits derived from their correction
1999	Edwin Sarver	San Antonio, TX	Modeling Optic Corrections
1982	Morton Sarver*	Berkeley, California	Contact lens effects upon the anatomy and physiology of the eye
2005	Steven Schallhorn	San Diego, California	What have we learned about vision correction through refractive surgery in aviators?
2005	Debra Schaumberg	Boston, Massachusetts	Contact lens wear and dry eye syndromes
2001	Oliver Schein*	Baltimore, Maryland	Measuring vision-related QOL: Importance of the patient perspective
1990	Dinesh Shah	Gainesville, Florida	Lens Solution Interactions and Performance
1984	Dinesh Shah	Gainesville, Florida	Surface chemistry of the eye and contact lens
1995	James Sheedy	Berkeley, California	A visual quality integrator: visual task performance
1988	Jacob Sivak	Waterloo, Ontario Canada	Corneal Role in the Aberrations of the Eye
2003	Earl Smith*	Houston, Texas	Emmetropization: A vision-dependent process

1999	Gabor A. Somarjai*	Berkeley, California	Surface vibrational spectroscopy and atomic force microscopy studies of polymer and polymer blend interfaces with air, water, and protein solutions
2001	SP Srinivas	Bloomington, Indiana	The molecular response of the epithelium to mechanical forces
1995	Kenneth Taylor	Cambridge, Massachusetts	The excimer laser and its impact on your practice/ business
1999	Larry N. Thibos	Bloomington, Indiana	Wavefront measurement in spectacle, RGP, and soft contact lens wearers
1984	John Tiffany	Oxford, United Kingdom	Composition and property of tears
1997	Brian Tighe*	Birmingham, United Kingdom	The aqueous sandwich: Understanding the bread and butter. Understanding and modeling the corneal surface and superficial lipid layer that "sandwich" the aqueous
1990	Brian Tighe*	Birmingham, United Kingdom	The Correlation of Structure with Properties and Properties with Performance
2001	Scheffer Tseng	Miami, Florida	Discomfort and dryness produced by CL wear
1997	Sally Twinning	Columbus, Ohio	Host and bacterial proteases in infection and inflammation
1995	Jean Weiner-Kronish	San Francisco, California	What can we learn from studies of pseudomonas aeruginosa lung infections about contact lens-related infections
1995	Mark Willcox*	Sydney, Australia	What we know-What are the critical unanswered questions?
2003	Christine Wildsoet	Berkeley, California	Myopia control: Pharmacological options and treatment issues

1999	David Williams	Rochester, New York	Evaluating multifocal contact lenses with wavefront sensing
1993	Graeme Wilson*	Birmingham, Alabama	Tissue responses to contact Jenses and refractive surgery: an overview of the field
1988	Graeme Wilson*	Birmingham, Alabama	Epithelial Desquamation And Contact Lens Wear
1997	Steven Wilson*	Cleveland, Ohio	Contact lenses and the ocular surface cytokines and potential effects on corneal structure
1993	Steven Wilson*	Dallas, Texas	Triumphs and horizons in the analysis of corneal topography

(ISCLR members designated by an *)

Appendix 8

Honorary Life/Emeritus Members

Irving Borish
Hikaru Hamano
Antonio Henriquez
Robert Koetting
Richard Pearson
Pierre Rocher
Montague Ruben (Founding President)
Otto Wichterle (Patron)

Appendix 9

Otto Wichterle Biographical Summary*

WICHTERLE, Otto, Dr tech, DSc academician. *PA* Senior scientific worker (Czechoslovak Academy of Sciences) and consultant for contact lenses (Spofa Pharmaceutical Works, Prague). *EPA* Institute of Technology, Technical University, Prague (1931-35). DSc, 1936. Charles University, Faculty of Medicine, 1935-38. Assistant lecturer, Institute for Experimental Organic Chemistry, Technical University, Prague, 1935-39. Expelled by Nazis from the University, 1939. Research Institute, Bata, Zlin, Head of Polymer Department, 1942-43 and 1944-45. Gestapo prison, 1942-43. Assistant Professor of Organic Chemistry, Chemical Faculty. Technical University of Prague, 1945. Chemical Consultant to Slovac Chemical Industry, 1946-49. Assistant Professor, Organic Chemistry, Charles Univer· sity, 1947. Professor, Macromolecular Chemistry and Technology, Technical University, Prague, 1949 to present. Dean, Technical University, Faculty of Organic Technology, 1953. State Prize for Chemistry, 1953. Head, Department for Macromolecular Chem· istry, Chemical Institute, Czechoslovak Academy of Sciences, 1955. Scientific Secretary, Chemical Section, Czechoslovak Academy of Sciences, 1954. Regular Member (Academician) Czechoslovak Academv of Sciences, 1956. Chairman, Commission for Macromolecular Chemistry, Czechoslovak Academy of Sciences, 1956. Director. Institute of Macromolecular Chemistry, Czechoslovak Academy of Sciences, Prague, 1959. IUPAC (International Union of Pure and Applied Chemistry) Bureau H-1970 member, 1962 to date. IUPAC Titular Member, 1963 to present. Chairman, IUPAC Macromolecular Commission, 1965. Vice-Chairman, Scientific Board of Theory of Chemical Processes of the Czechoslovak Academy of Science, 1963 to present. State Prize, 1967 (hydrophilic gels). Member, IUPAC Executive Committee, 1967. President, IUPAC Macromolecular Division, 1967 to present. Member, ad hoc Committee for Inter-disciplinary Matters, IUPAC, 1969-70. Member, German Academy of Science, Berlin, 1967. Member, Czechoslovak

National Council, 1968·69. Member, Czechoslovak Federal Parliament, 1968-69. President, Organising Committee, Society for Human Rights, 1968. President, Union of Czech Scien· tific Workers, 1969-70. Centennial Foreign Fellow. American Chemical Society, 1976. Javal Award, Tokyo. 1978. *LW Chemistry* (general, organic and macromolecular): 6 books. over 100 publi· cations in scientific journals. Over 150 patents. Contact lenses: Numerous publications in professional and scientific journals. 42 patents including basic inventions of soft lenses (lathe cutting pro· cess, 1963; spincasting process. 1961). *HA* U Andelky 27,162.00 Prague 6. *OA* Institute of Macromolecular Chemistry, 162.06 Prague 6. Czechoslovakia.

*   Reprinted from International Optical &ear Book and Diary, Reed Business Publishing, Surrey England, 1983

Appendix 10

*Ruben Biographical Summary***

RUBEN, Montague, MED.Y, CIRUG (University of Barcelona), FRCS, FCOph, DOMS, LRCP. *PA* Formerly Distinguished Professor, Visual Science, University of Houston, USA; Past Director, Institute of Contact Lens Research, College of Optometry, Houston; Honorary Surgeon, Moorfields Eye Hospital 1983-; Past Visiting Professor, Optometry Department, The City University; Clinical Teacher in Ophthalmology, Faculty of Medicine, University of London; Past Chairman, Whitley Council (Hospital Opticians Section) Management side; Member, Committee of Surgical and Dental Materials (DHSS); Chairman, Sub-Committee Ophthalmic Preparations (DHSS); Past President, British Medical Contact Lens Society; Past President, Contact Lens Society, Great Britain; Past President, International Society for Contact Lens Research 1980-82; Liveryman, Society of Apothecaries. *EPA* Honorary Editor, various journals, *LW* 200 scientific papers. Chapters in May & Worth, "Practical Orthoptics" and "Corneal-Plastic Surgery", Books-"Clinical Optics-Diagnostic Outline", "Contact Lens Practice" (Bailliere Tindall, 1974), "Understanding Contact Lenses" (Heinemann, 1976), "Soft Contact Lenses" (J.Wiley, New York, 1979), "Revision, Clinical Optics" (MacMillan, 1981) and "Atlas of Contact Lens Practice" (Woolfe Publications, 1983), 2nd edition 1989, "Contact Lenses"-Hamano & Ruben (Donitz 1986), "Diagnostic Pictures in Ophthalmology"-Ruben 1987 (Wolfe Med. Atlas), "Your Eyes and Their Care"-Ruben and Wintle (Granada 1986), "Medical Aspects of Contact Lenses", published P.G. Press, Singapore, by Ruben & Khoo 1989, In preparation with M. Guillon, I. Fatt and S. Harris, "Modern Contact Lens Practice", publishers. Chapman & Hall "Contact Lenses (Scientific Aspects)" with M Guillon. in press Chapman & Hall. *OA* 20 Sevenstones Drive, Broadstairs, Kent CT10 lTW. *Hobbies:* Painting, music.

** Reprinted from International Optical &ear Book and Diary, Reed Business Publishing, Surrey England, 1994

Appendix 11

*Graduate Student Symposium Presenters**

2007	Amanda Ackerman	UC-Berkeley	Berkeley, California	Corneal epithelial cells eat and kill bacteria, but Pseudomonas can evade this. A novel defense mechanism of the corneal surface: Killing of internalized bacteria by corneal epithelial cells.
2007	Irania Alarcon	UC-Berkeley	Berkeley, California	In vivo factors that impact corneal epithelial resistance to bacterial penetration
2007	Jennifer Choo	Pacific University	Forest Grove, Oregon	Orthokeratology progressive and regressive corneal changes: A histological study
2007	Katie Edwards	Vision CRC	Sydney, Australia	Risk factors for contact lens related microbial keratitis in Australia
2007	Paul Gifford	Vision CRC	Sydney, Australia	Time course for topographic changes in the 1st week of overnight hyperopic OK
2007	Maud Gorbet	Waterloo & McMaster University	Canada	Corneal epithelial cell viability and integrin expression is affected by contact lens packaging solutions

2007	Santosh Khanal	Glasgow Caledonian University	Glasgow, UK	Comparison between tear hyperosmolarity and ocular surface tests in assessing tear dynamics
2007	Nancy Kier	School of Optometry	Waterloo, Canada	Clinical impact of pre-soaking a silicone hydrogel in a MPS care solution on a group of systematic wearers
2007	Ajay Kumar	University of New South Wales	Sydney, Australia	Guinea pig model of contact lens acute red eye and/or infiltrative keratitis response
2007	Holly Lorentz	School of Optometry	Waterloo, Canada	In vitro deposition of lipid onto contact lens materials can lower contact angle wettability of surface-modified silicone hydrogel contact lens materials
2007	Dimitra Makrynioti	University of Manchester	Manchester, UK	Variations in corneal morphology across the cornea: A study in normal subjects and contact lens wearers
2007	Jose Meijome	University of Minho	Braha, Portugal	In vitro dehydration of conventional and silicone hydrogel contact lenses
2007	Rachael Peterson	School of Optometry	Waterloo, Canada	Objective measures of changes in corneal staining
2007	Ruby Prakasan	LV Prasad Eye Inst, Vision CRC	Sydney, Australia	Development of corneal iron ring deposits with corneal inlays
2007	Danielle Robertson	UT Southwestern Medical Center	Dallas, Texas	Molecular mediators of corneal epithelial homeostasis
2007	Ulrike Stahl	Vision CRC	Sydney, Australia	The influence of temporary collagen inserts on ocular comfort and contact lens osmolality during contact lens wear
2007	Lakshman Subbaraman	University of Waterloo	Waterloo, Canada	Activity of lysozyme deposited on conventional and silicone hydrogel contact lens materials as a function of time

2005	Jennifer Choo	Pacific University	Forest Grove, Oregon	Optical modeling of corneal shape with orthokeratology, The ideal shape of the cornea after orthokeratology
2005	Tim Conibear	University of New South Wales	Sydney, Australia	Characterization of protease IV as a virulence determinant in clinical ocular isolates of Pseudomonas aeruginosa
2005	Blanka Golebiowski	University of New South Wales	Sydney, Australia	Symptoms in low and high Dk/T soft contact lens wear
2005	Susan Hiemer	Harvard Medical School	Boston, Massachusetts	Staphyloccocus aureus alters cytokine release from corneal epithelial cells, Toxigenic Stahylococcus aureus downregulates proinflammatory cytokine release from cultured human corneal epithelial cells
2005	Jessica Horne	UH College of Optometry	Houston, Texas	Is tissue loss the cause of ectasia in pathologically and iatrogenically thinned corneas?
2005	Lisa Keay	University of New South Wales	Sydney, Australia	Factors influencing the severity of contact lens-related keratitis
2005	Pete Kollbaum	Indiana University	Bloomington, Indiana	Impact of contact lens decentrations on the correction of optical aberrations
2005	Ajay Kumar	University of New South Wales	Sydney, Australia	An animal model for bacterial induced inflammation during contact lens wear
2005	Anisa Mahomed	Aston University	Birmingham, UK	Friction and lubricity measurement: Effects of lens wear
2005	Inna Maltseva	School of Optometry	Berkeley, California	Contact lens wear suppresses innate defenses of corneal epithelial cells, Contact lens wear in vitro compromises human corneal epithelial cell innate defense responses against bacteria

2005	Aisling Mann	Aston University	Birmingham, UK	Kinin activity in contact lens wear
2005	Danielle Robertson	UT Southwestern Medical Center	Dallas, Texas	A new tissue-engineered human corneal epithelium: Differentiative and regenerative potential
2005	Garreth Ross	Aston University	Birmingham, England	Surface modification by macromolecular entrapment, Comfort enhancement by macromolecular entrapment: Understanding the mechanism
2005	Ping Situ	University of Waterloo	Waterloo, Canada	The relationship between corneal and conjunctival sensitivity dry eye symptoms, tear film stability and ocular surface characteristics
2005	Tracey Shubert	Vision CRC	Sydney, Australia	Antibacterial and immunological effect of furanone-based antibacterials
2005	Cheryl Skotnitsky	Vision CRC	Sydney, Australia	Etiology of local contact lens—induced papillary conjunctivitis in recurrent events
2005	Ulrike Stahl	Vision CRC	Sydney, Australia	Influences of osmotic factors in contact lens comfort
2005	Lakshman Subbarraman	University of Waterloo	Waterloo, Canada	Part 2 contact lens dry eye: Kinetics of 125-I—labelled lysozyme deposition on silicone hydrogel FDA Group II and Group IV contact lenses
2003	BMK Bandara	University of New South Wales	Sydney, Australia	Salicylic acid
2003	Tim Conibear	University of New South Wales	Sydney, Australia	quorum sensing
2003	Blanka Golebiowski	University of New South Wales	Sydney, Australia	Symptomatology during transition from low to high Dk/t soft contact lens wear and its association with ocular surface sensitivity

Year	Name	Institution	Location	Title
2003	Ying Guo	IU School of Optometry	Bloomington, Indiana	
2003	Isabelle Jalbert	University of New South Wales	Sydney, Australia	Effect of lenses on corneal epithelium
2003	Thomas John			Multivariate factors associated with corneal infiltrative events in extended soft contact lens wearers
2003	Thai Leechoon			Recovery of the tear film from contact lens wear
2003	Tracy Nguyen	IU School of Optometry	Bloomington, Indiana	Does barrier integrity and epithelial energy metabolism change in overnight orthokeratology?
2003	Cheryl Skotnitksy	Vision CRC	Sydney, Australia	Recurrence of contact lens induced papillary conjunctivitis (CLPC) in high Dk silicone hydrogel lenses
2003	Jalaiah Varikooty	University of Waterloo	Waterloo, Canada	Ocular surface heating alters bulbar redness
2001	Ahmed Alharbi	University of New South Wales	Sydney, Australia	Overnight orthokeratology induces central epithelial thinning
2001	Geoffrey Brent	University of New South Wales	Sydney, Australia	Finite element modeling of closed eye pressure under a 3-D axisymmetric SCL and comparison with clinical outcomes
2001	Susan Han	UC College of Optomery	Berkeley, California	Changes in post-lens tear film thickness over a seven hour wear period
2001	Patrick Ladage	UT Ophthal&UH Optometry	Houston, Texas	Recovery time of epithelial proliferation rate in the rabbit cornea following 24-hours of low 02 RGP lens wear
2001	Meng Lin	UC School of Optometry	Berkeley, California	Ethnicity effects—tear mixing
2001	David Miles			Apoptosis of the epithelial cells of the ocular surface

2001	Kimberley Miller	UC School of Optometry	Berkeley, California	Fenestrations and tear mixing efficiency
2001	Kelly Nichols	College of Optometry	Columbus, Ohio	Quality of life in dry eye patients
2001	Cheryl Skotnitsky	University of New South Wales	Sydney, Australia	Factors associated with contact lens induced papillary conjunctivitis (CLPC)
2001	Mary Stanley	UC Dept of Chemical Engineering	Berkeley, California	A model eye to validate dispersive tear mixing
2001	Jalaiah Varikooty	University of Waterloo	Waterloo, Canada	Ocular discomfort upon tear drying—a semi-continuous method to simultaneously rate the qualitative and quantitative dimensions of discomfort
2001	Jay Wang	University of Waterloo	Waterloo, Canada	Tear film thickness measured with optical coherence tomography
1999	Marcella Browne	University of New South Wales	Sydney, Australia	UV Based Methods for Improved Contact Lens Surfaces
1999	Anuj Chauhan	School of Optometry UC	Berkeley, California	Modeling Lens Motion
1999	James Doshi	University of Texas Health Science Center	San Antonio, TX	Models Predict Actual Visual Performance
1999	Victoria Evans	University of New South Wales	Sydney, Australia	The Effect of Phosphodiesterase Inhibitors on the Tear Film
1999	Melissa Glasson	University of New South Wales	Sydney, Australia	Dryness Symptoms and Contact Lens Wear
1999	Xin Hong	IU School of Optometry	Bloomington, Indiana	Optical Effects of Drying Soft Contact Lenses
1999	Carol Lakkis	University of Melbourne	Melbourne, Australia	Contact Lens Disinfection Enhances the Survival of Cytotoxic P.aeruginosa Stains
1999	Ellen Lee	UC-Berkeley	Berkeley, California	Cell Killing by Cytotoxic P.aeruginosa

1999	Meng Lin	UC-Berkeley	Berkeley, California	Effects of Oxygen Permeability of RGP's on Epithelial Barrier Function Can the Layer between the Lens and the Cornea be Measured
1999	Fiona Lydon	Biomaterials Research Institute	Birmingham, UK	Why Do Contact Lenses Adhere to the Corneal Surface
1999	Carole Maldonado-Codina	UMIST	Manchester, UK	In Vivo Confocal Microscopy of the Cornea Following Extended Wear of Acuvue vs Silicone Hydrogel Contact Lenses
1999	Aisling Mann	Aston University	Birmingham, England	The Impact of Daily Disposability on the Deposition of Immunoregulatory Proteins
1999	Sally McArthur	University of New South Wales	Sydney, Australia	Surface—MALDI—MS Analysis of In Vivo Contact Lens Protein
1999	Arti Shah	UC-Berkeley	Berkeley, California	A Pilot Study of Corneal Surface Flora
1999	Archana Thakur	University of New South Wales	Sydney, Australia	Immunity of P.aeruginosa Keratitis in Rats
1999	Vicky Vallas	University of New South Wales	Sydney, Australia	Bacterial Invasion of Ocular Mucosal Surfaces
1997	Jing Jing Bi	Commonwealth Scientific and Industrial Research Organization	Victoria, Australia	A potential contact lens laminate: A polymer with outstanding Dk and an ultrathin hydrophilic coating
1997	Qian Garrett	University of New South Wales	Sydney, Australia	Effect of hydrogel lens monomer constituents
1997	Emma Hume	University of New South Wales	Sydney, Australia	The production of microbial keratitis or contact lens induced acute red eye is dependent on the type of bacteria that colonize the contact lens and not on the contact lens wearer

1997	Jenny Lan	University of New South Wales	Sydney, Australia	The effect of tear secretory IgA on PMN cells recruitment in eye closure environment
1997	Ellen Lee	UC-Berkeley	Berkeley, California	Mechanism of corneal cell killing by intracellular pseudomonas aeriginosa
1997	Nancy McNamara	UC-San Francisco	San Francisco, California	Tear replenishment rates under soft contact lenses, Extended wear affects epithelial permeability
1997	Ian Pearce	Glasgow Caledonian University	Glasgow, Scotland	Tear dynamics and the compartmentalization of the tear film
1997	Maxine Tan	University of New South Wales	Sydney, Australia	Matching sensations of contact lens wear with known stimuli
1995	Nerida Cole	University of New South Wales	Sydney, Australia	Cytokines in the anterior eye
1995	Brigitte Cowell	UC-Berkeley	Berkeley, California	Physiological effects on surface properties of pseudomonas aeruginosa
1995	Valerie Franklin	Aston University	Birmingham, UK	Fluorescence spectroscopic characterization of worn contact lenses
1995	Emma Hume	University of New South Wales	Sydney, Australia	Contact lens associated serratia marcescens and its interaction with the host defense mechanism
1995	Peter Kingshott	Commonwealth Scientific and Industrial Research Organization	Victoria, Australia	XPS and TOF-SSIMS characterization of soft lens fouling
1995	Jenny Lan	University of New South Wales	Sydney, Australia	Bacterial specific IgA in human tears
1995	Carol Leitch	University of New South Wales	Sydney, Australia	Identification and enumeration of staphylococci isolated from disposable soft contact lenses

1995	Jerry Paugh	Southern California College of Optometry	Fullerton, California	Measurement of tear vehicles and artificial tears and potentially, tear viscosity in situ
1995	Nancy McNamara	University of California	San Francisco, California	The effects of elevated blood glucose on corneal structure and function
1995	Timothy Williams			The effect of conditioning films on bacterial adhesion to contact lenses
1995	Steven Wiffen	Mayo Clinic	Rochester, Minnesota	Central and peripheral corneal endothelial cell density and morphology in normals and contact lens wearers
1993	Michael S Conners	New York Medical College	Valhalla, New York	Cytochrome P450-derived arachidonic acid metabolites in the corneal epithelium: novel inflammatory mediator, Complications of contact lens wear are alleviated by manipulation of corneal cytochrome P450
1993	Charline Gauthier	University of New South Wales	Sydney, Australia	Epithelial changes following PRK
1993	John Laurent	University of Alabama at Birmingham	Birmingham, Alabama	The role of basal cell migration in maintaining epithelial integrity
1993	Naoyuki Maeda	LSU Eye Center	New Orleans, Louisiana	Automated keratoconus detection for refractive surgery and contact lens candidates using corneal topography
1993	Philip Morgan	UMIST	Manchester, UK	Assessment of the tear film by ocular thermography
1993	Marta Portoles	Schepens Eye Research Institute	Boston, Massachusetts	A new approach for the prevention of bacterial keratitis: adhesive polymers
1990	Suzanne Fleizsig	University of Melbourne	Melbourne, Australia	Adherence of pseudomonas aeruginosa to human corneal epithelial cells

1990	Fiona Stapleton	University of New South Wales	Sydney, Australia	Electron microscopy of bacterial biofilm
1990	Helen Swarbrick	University of New South Wales	Sydney, Australia	The etiology of RGP lens adherence
1986	Hans Bleshoy		London, UK	Ultrastructure of nerves in keratoconic and normal corneas
1986	Joseph Bonano	University of California	Berkeley, California	In vivo measurement of human corneal stromal pH.
1986	Arthur Ho	University of New South Wales	Sydney, Australia	Effect of overnight and daily wear of HGP and SCL on epithelial permeability.
1986	Steven Kwok	University of New South Wales	Sydney, Australia	Free-swelling properties of the normal and healed cat corneal stroma.

* Due to the paucity of records, sponsored graduate students going to symposia before 1990 are not fully included.

Appendix 12

Symposium Corporate Sponsors

3M Vision Care
Advanced Medical Optics
Alcon Laboratories Inc./Alcon Medical
Allergan (Inc/ Optical/ Pharmaceuticals)
Allergan-Hydron
Aspect Visioncare / Coopervision
Bausch & Lomb
Biocompatibles Eyecare/International
CIBA Vision Corporation
Clearlab
Cooper Vision
Eye Sys
International Hydron, Inc
Johnson & Johnson Vision Care Inc./Vistakon
Menicon Co. Ltd.
Ocular Sciences Inc
Paragon Vision Sciences
Polymer Technology Corporation
Pilkington
Ross Laboratories
Sola Barnes-Hind / Sola Syntex

Bibliography

Barr, J. (2005). History and development of contact lenses. In E. S. Bennett, & B. A. Weissman, *Clinical Contact Lens Practice.* Philadelphia: Lipincott Williams & Willkins.

Dreifus, M. (1978). The development of pHEMA of contact lens wear. In M. Ruben, *Soft contact lenses : clinical and applied technology* (pp. 7-16). New York: John Wiley & Son.

Efron, N. (2002). *Contact Lens Practice.* Oxford: Butterworth Heinmann.

Hudlicky, M. (1998). My Reminiscences of Professor Otto Wichterle. *The Chemical Educator, 3* (6), pp. 1-8.

International Optical Year Book and Diary. (1983). Sutton, Surrey(UK): Reed.

Koetting, R. A. (Director). (1990). *Living history of contact lenses. #26 (Fatt and Wichterle)* [Motion Picture], from American Optometric Association, St. Louis, MO.

Mandel, R. B. (1988). *Contact Lens Practice. Charles Thomas. Springfield (IL).*

Pearson, R. M. Otto Wichterle: October 27, 1913-August 18, 1998. *British Contact Lens Association. Presentation on October 8, 2008.*

Phillips, A. J., Speedwell, L., Stone, J., & Hough, T. (1997). *Contact Lenses. Butterworth Heinemann*

Ruben, M. (1982). *Color atlas of contact lenses & prosthetics.* Connecticut: Appleton-Century-Crofts.

Ruben, M. (1975). *Contact Lens Practice; Visual, Therapeutic and Prosthetic.* London: Cassell & Collier Macmillan Publishers Ltd.

Ruben, M. (1978). *Soft Contact Lenses: Clinical and Applied Technology.* John Wiley & Sons.

Sweeney, D. F. (2004). *Silicone hydrogels : continuous-wear contact lenses. Butterworth-Heinemann, 2nd Edition*

Wichterle O, L. D. (1961). *Patent No. 2 976575.* USA.

Wichterle, O. L. (1960). Hydrophil gels for biological use. *Nature, 185,* pp. 117-118.

Wichterle, O. (1994). *Recollections.* Prague: IDEU REPRO.

Wichterle, O. (1978). The Beginning of the Soft Lens. In M. Ruben, *Soft Contact Lenses.* New York: Wiley.